Pelvic Floor Disorders

A Woman's Guide to Pelvic Floor Health and Recovery

Ethan D. Anderson

Xspurts.com

A New Zealand Designed Product

Other Versions Available

Why limit yourself to just one format?

This book is now available in physical, digital, and audiobook options.

Choose the way you love to read and dive into the story today. You won't regret it!

Digital ISBN: 9781776969456
Physical ISBN: 9781776969449
Audio ISBN:

To obtain a different format of this book at a discounted price, please get in touch with us at:

http://isbn.xspurts.com/

Contents

Have Questions / Comments?

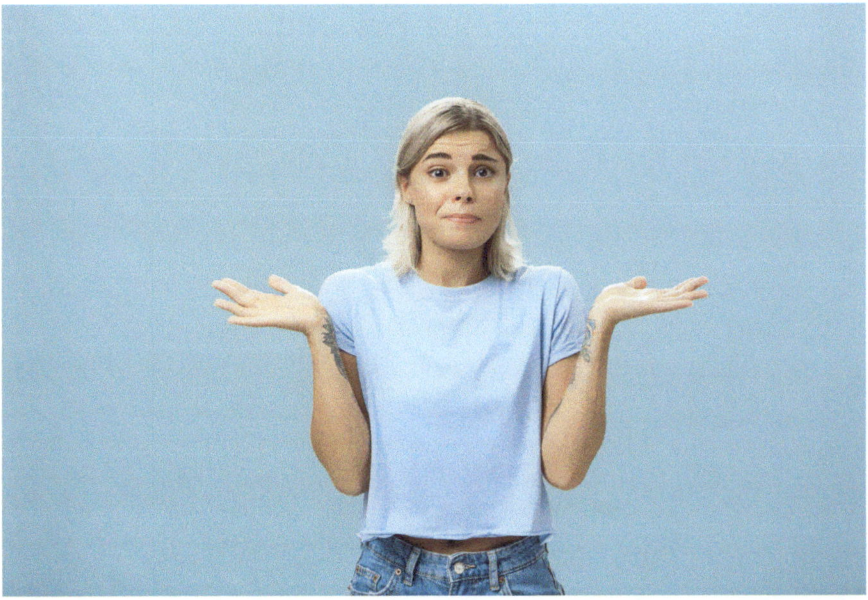

This book was designed to cover as much information as possible, but I know I have probably missed something, or some new amazing discovery has just come out.

If you notice something missing or have a question that I failed to answer, please get in touch and let me know. If I can, I will email you an answer and also update the book so others can also benefit from it.

Thanks For Being Awesome :)

Submit Your Questions / Comments At:

https://questions.xspurts.com

Get Free Stuff

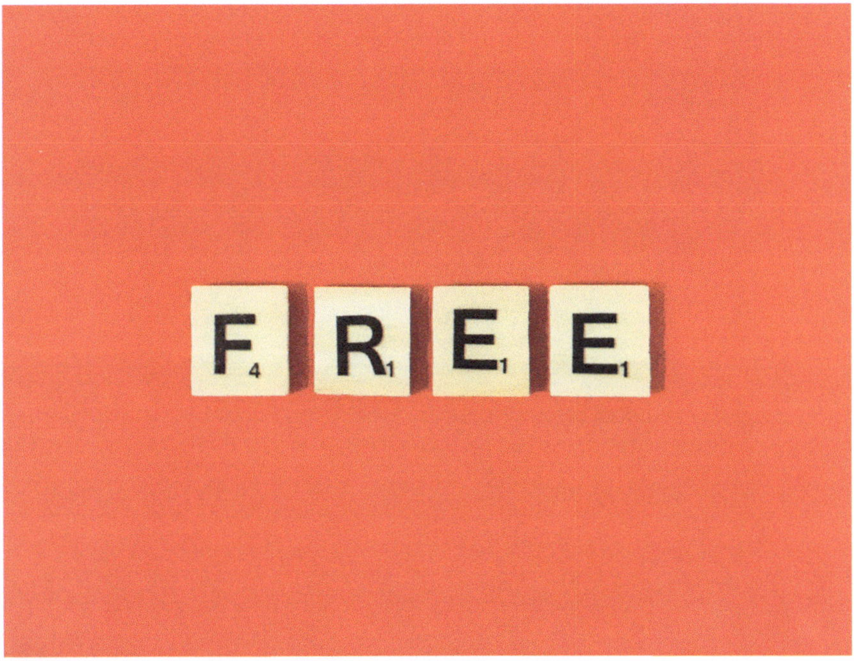

We love writing and have produced a huge number of books.

For being one of our amazing readers, we would love to offer you more books we have created, 100% free.

To claim this limited time special offer, simply go to the site below and enter your name and email address.

You will then receive loads (as we love our readers so much :) of our great books, content and audio direct to your email account, 100% free!

Get Loads of FREE Stuff at:

https://free.xspurts.com

Chapter One

Introduction to the Pelvic Floor

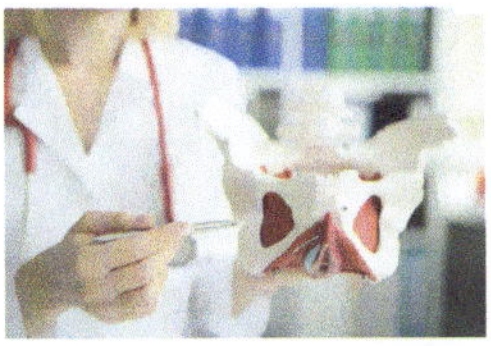

The pelvic floor is a group of muscles, ligaments, and tissues that form a sling-like structure at the bottom of the pelvis. It supports the pelvic organs, including the bladder, uterus, and rectum, and helps control urinary and fecal continence. The pelvic floor muscles also play a key role in sexual function and are important for childbirth.

While the pelvic floor is essential for our overall health and well-being, it often goes overlooked and is rarely discussed. In fact, many people are not aware of the importance of maintaining a healthy pelvic floor until they experience problems, such as incontinence or pelvic pain.

This book aims to provide an in-depth look at pelvic floor health and disorders, covering topics such as exercises to strengthen the pelvic floor, common pelvic floor disorders, and treatment options. Whether you are experiencing pelvic floor problems or simply want to maintain a healthy pelvic floor, this book is a valuable resource for understanding and improving your pelvic floor health.

Chapter Two

What is a Pelvic Floor?

The pelvic floor is a group of muscles and tissues that form a sling-like structure in the pelvis, supporting the pelvic organs such as the bladder, uterus, and rectum.

The pelvic floor muscles attach to the front, back, and sides of the pelvic bone and work together to control the opening and closing of the urethra, anus, and vagina in women.

In men, the pelvic floor muscles support the bladder and rectum, and control the flow of urine and semen.

The pelvic floor also plays a vital role in sexual function and childbirth.

When the pelvic floor is functioning correctly, it provides stability and support for the pelvic organs, prevents urinary and fecal incontinence, and contributes to sexual pleasure.

The pelvic floor is an essential part of the body's core musculature and helps stabilize the trunk and hips during movement. Like other muscles in the body, the pelvic floor can become weak or injured, leading to a variety of pelvic floor disorders.

Chapter Three

Importance of pelvic floor health

The pelvic floor is an integral part of the body, and its health is crucial for both men and women. This network of muscles, tissues, and ligaments is responsible for supporting the bladder, uterus, and rectum, as well as maintaining bowel and bladder control. The pelvic floor muscles are also essential for sexual function and pleasure.

When the pelvic floor muscles are weakened, it can result in a range of complications, including urinary incontinence, fecal incontinence, pelvic organ prolapse, and sexual dysfunction. These issues can have a significant impact on an individual's quality of life and self-esteem.

Therefore, it is essential to maintain a healthy pelvic floor to prevent these complications from arising. This can be achieved through various exercises and lifestyle changes, such as Kegels and maintaining a healthy weight. By keeping the pelvic floor strong and healthy, individuals can improve their overall wellbeing and avoid potential complications.

Chapter Four

Functions of the pelvic floor

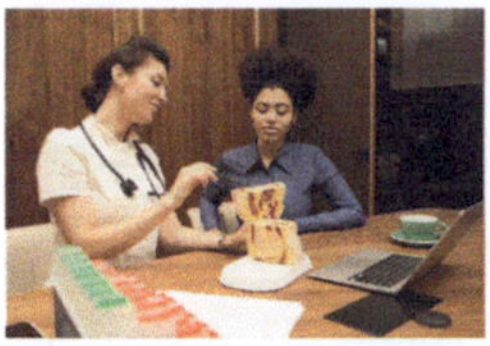

The pelvic floor is responsible for a number of essential functions that are crucial for our overall health and well-being. These functions include:

Support: The pelvic floor muscles provide support to the pelvic organs such as the bladder, uterus, and rectum. They keep these organs in their proper place and prevent them from dropping down or prolapsing.

Control: The pelvic floor muscles are responsible for controlling the opening and closing of the urethra, anus, and vagina. They play a vital role in maintaining continence, or the ability to control urine and bowel movements.

Sexual function: The pelvic floor muscles are also involved in sexual function, both in men and women. They help to maintain penile and clitoral erections and control ejaculation. In women, they also contribute to vaginal lubrication and orgasm.

Core stability: The pelvic floor muscles are part of the core muscle group that stabilizes the trunk and pelvis. They work together with the deep abdominal and back muscles to provide a stable base for movement and to protect the spine.

Overall, the pelvic floor is a vital part of our body and its health is essential to our overall well-being.

Chapter Five

The anatomy of the pelvic floor

The pelvic floor is a group of muscles, ligaments, and tissues that form a hammock-like structure in the pelvic area. It supports the pelvic organs, which include the bladder, uterus, and rectum. The pelvic floor muscles are also responsible for controlling the passage of urine, feces, and gas.

The pelvic floor muscles can be divided into three layers:

Superficial layer: The superficial layer consists of the bulbocavernosus and ischiocavernosus muscles, which surround the vagina in women and the base of the penis in men.

Middle layer: The middle layer includes the pubococcygeus, iliococcygeus, and puborectalis muscles. These muscles form a sling-like structure that supports the pelvic organs.

Deep layer: The deep layer consists of the levator ani muscles, which attach to the pubic bone at the front of the pelvis and the coccyx at the back.

The pelvic floor muscles work in coordination with the abdominal and back muscles to maintain posture, support the spine, and control bowel and bladder function.

It's important to note that the pelvic floor can weaken over time due to factors such as pregnancy, childbirth, aging, obesity, and certain medical conditions. This weakening can lead to pelvic floor disorders, which can affect quality of life and daily functioning. In the following chapters, we will discuss common pelvic floor disorders, their causes, symptoms, and treatment options.

Chapter Six

The causes of pelvic floor dysfunction

The pelvic floor is a complex system of muscles, ligaments, and tissues that work together to support the bladder, uterus, rectum, and other pelvic organs. Pelvic floor dysfunction occurs when this system is weakened, damaged, or compromised in some way. There are several causes of pelvic floor dysfunction, including:

1. Pregnancy and childbirth: The process of carrying a baby to term and giving birth can put a significant amount of strain on the pelvic floor. This can result in weakened or damaged muscles, which can cause problems with incontinence, pelvic pain, and other issues.

2. Aging: As we age, our muscles and tissues naturally lose some of their strength and elasticity. This can cause the pelvic floor to weaken over time, leading to problems with incontinence and other symptoms.

3. Chronic constipation: Straining to have a bowel movement can put pressure on the pelvic floor muscles and cause them to weaken over time.

4. Chronic coughing: Like constipation, chronic coughing can put pressure on the pelvic floor and cause it to weaken.

5. Obesity: Being overweight can put additional strain on the pelvic

floor muscles and lead to dysfunction.

6. Certain medical conditions: Medical conditions such as endometriosis, pelvic organ prolapse, and pelvic inflammatory disease can all contribute to pelvic floor dysfunction.

7. Certain surgical procedures: Surgeries that involve the pelvic area, such as a hysterectomy, can damage the pelvic floor muscles and lead to dysfunction.

It's important to note that some people may be more prone to pelvic floor dysfunction than others due to genetics or other factors. Additionally, some people may experience pelvic floor dysfunction without an identifiable cause.

Chapter Seven

Common Pelvic Floor Disorders

Pelvic floor disorders are conditions that affect the muscles, ligaments, and tissues that support the pelvic organs. These disorders are common, affecting millions of women and men around the world. Here are some of the most common pelvic floor disorders:

1. Urinary incontinence: This is a common condition that affects both men and women, and it is characterized by the involuntary leakage of urine. There are two types of urinary incontinence: stress incontinence, which occurs when there is pressure on the bladder, and urge incontinence, which is caused by an overactive bladder.

2. Pelvic organ prolapse: This occurs when the pelvic organs (bladder, uterus, or rectum) shift from their normal position and bulge into the vaginal wall. Pelvic organ prolapse can cause discomfort, pain, and urinary incontinence.

3. Fecal incontinence: This is the involuntary leakage of fecal matter. It is often caused by damage to the anal sphincter muscles or the nerves that control them.

4. Chronic pelvic pain: This is pain that lasts for six months or longer in the pelvic area. Chronic pelvic pain can be caused by a variety of conditions, including endometriosis, pelvic inflammatory disease, and irritable bowel syndrome.

5. Sexual dysfunction: Pelvic floor disorders can cause sexual dysfunction, such as pain during sex or difficulty achieving orgasm.

It is important to note that pelvic floor disorders can affect both men and women, but they are more common in women. Pregnancy and childbirth, menopause, and certain medical conditions (such as obesity and chronic constipation) can increase the risk of developing pelvic floor disorders.

Urinary incontinence

Urinary incontinence is a common pelvic floor disorder that affects people of all ages, genders, and backgrounds. It occurs when the muscles and tissues that support the bladder and urethra are weakened or damaged, causing a loss of bladder control.

There are different types of urinary incontinence, including:

Stress incontinence: This occurs when physical activities such as coughing, sneezing, laughing, or lifting cause a sudden increase in intra-abdominal pressure, which pushes down on the bladder and results in urine leakage.

Urge incontinence: This occurs when there is a sudden and strong urge to urinate, and the bladder muscles contract involuntarily, causing urine to leak before reaching the toilet.

Mixed incontinence: This is a combination of stress and urge incontinence.

Overflow incontinence: This occurs when the bladder is unable to empty completely, causing a continuous dribbling of urine.

Functional incontinence: This is a type of incontinence that is caused by physical or mental disabilities that prevent a person from reaching the toilet in time.

Urinary incontinence can have a significant impact on a person's quality of life, causing embarrassment, anxiety, and social isolation. Fortunately, there are many treatment options available that can help manage or even cure urinary incontinence.

Fecal incontinence

Fecal incontinence is the inability to control bowel movements, resulting in stool leakage or unintentional bowel movements. It is a common condition that affects people of all ages but is more prevalent in older adults and women. Fecal incontinence can cause embarrassment and affect a person's quality of life, making it difficult to participate in everyday activities.

The pelvic floor muscles are responsible for controlling bowel movements, and any weakness or damage to these muscles can result in fecal incontinence. The most common causes of fecal incontinence include damage to the muscles and nerves in the pelvic floor due to childbirth, injury, surgery, or aging. Other conditions that can contribute to fecal incontinence include diarrhea, constipation, inflammatory bowel disease, and certain medications.

Symptoms of fecal incontinence may include a strong urge to have a bowel movement, leakage of stool during physical activity, the sensation of incomplete bowel movements, and an inability to control bowel movements. Diagnosis of fecal incontinence involves a physical exam, medical history, and tests such as anal manometry, defecography, or anorectal ultrasonography.

Treatment for fecal incontinence may include pelvic floor exercises, dietary changes, medication, biofeedback therapy, or surgery in severe cases. Prevention of fecal incontinence includes maintaining a healthy diet, regular exercise, avoiding constipation, and avoiding or treating any underlying medical conditions.

Pelvic organ prolapse

Pelvic organ prolapse is a common pelvic floor disorder that occurs when one or more of the pelvic organs, such as the bladder, uterus, or rectum, descend into the vagina. This can be caused by weakened pelvic floor muscles and ligaments that are unable to support the organs properly.

Some common risk factors for pelvic organ prolapse include pregnancy and childbirth, menopause, and aging. Women who have given birth vaginally, have had a hysterectomy, or have a chronic cough or constipation may be at a higher risk of developing pelvic organ prolapse.

Symptoms of pelvic organ prolapse can include a feeling of pressure or heaviness in the pelvis, a bulge or protrusion felt in the vagina, urinary incontinence, and difficulty with bowel movements. Some women may not experience any symptoms at all.

Treatment options for pelvic organ prolapse vary depending on the severity of the condition and the symptoms experienced. In mild cases, exercises to strengthen the pelvic floor muscles may be enough to improve symptoms. For more severe cases, surgery may be necessary to lift and support the organs back into their proper position.

Pain during intercourse

Pain during intercourse, also known as dyspareunia, is a common pelvic floor disorder affecting both men and women. Dyspareunia can be experienced as a burning or aching sensation, and it can be caused by a variety of factors.

In women, dyspareunia may be caused by vaginal dryness, vaginal infections, vaginismus, endometriosis, pelvic inflammatory disease (PID), uterine prolapse, ovarian cysts, or fibroids. It can also be caused by scar tissue or adhesions resulting from surgery or childbirth. In some cases, the pain may be psychosomatic and caused by anxiety or other emotional factors.

In men, dyspareunia may be caused by prostatitis, Peyronie's disease, or other penile conditions. It can also be caused by nerve damage or muscle tension in the pelvic floor.

Treatment for dyspareunia will depend on the underlying cause. Treatment options may include physical therapy, medication, surgery, counseling, or other interventions. It is important to discuss any pain or discomfort during intercourse with a healthcare provider in order to determine the cause and appropriate treatment.

Pain in the pelvic area

Pelvic pain is a common problem that affects both men and women, and can have a significant impact on a person's quality of life. It can be a result of a variety of underlying causes, including pelvic floor dysfunction.

Pelvic pain can be described as pain or discomfort that is felt in the lower abdominal area, below the belly button, and above the legs. The pain can be constant or intermittent, and can range in severity from mild to severe. It can be a dull ache or a sharp, stabbing pain.

The causes of pelvic pain can vary widely, from injuries and infections to chronic medical conditions. In women, pelvic pain can be associated with gynecological problems such as endometriosis, ovarian cysts, and uterine fibroids. Men can also experience pelvic pain, which may be related to prostate problems or other conditions.

Pelvic pain can also be related to the muscles, ligaments, and nerves of the pelvic floor. Pelvic floor dysfunction can cause pain and discomfort in the pelvic area, as well as other symptoms such as urinary and fecal incontinence, and sexual dysfunction.

It is important to seek medical attention if you experience pelvic pain. Your healthcare provider can evaluate your symptoms and determine the underlying cause of your pain, and develop an appropriate treatment plan.

Urinary urgency and frequency

Urinary urgency and frequency are common symptoms of pelvic floor dysfunction. The pelvic floor muscles play an important role in maintaining urinary continence by supporting the bladder and urethra. When these muscles are weak, the bladder can become unstable and cause a sudden and urgent need to urinate.

Urinary frequency, or the need to urinate more often than usual, can also be a sign of pelvic floor dysfunction. This may be due to a weak or overactive bladder, or it may be caused by the muscles of the pelvic floor being unable to properly support the bladder.

Other symptoms that may be associated with urinary urgency and frequency include:

- Urinary incontinence
- Pain or discomfort during urination
- Difficulty starting or stopping urination

- Incomplete emptying of the bladder
- Blood in the urine

If you are experiencing urinary urgency and frequency, it is important to see a healthcare provider to determine the underlying cause and appropriate treatment. Treatment may involve pelvic floor muscle exercises, medication, or other interventions depending on the cause of the symptoms.

Constipation

Constipation is a common pelvic floor disorder that affects people of all ages, genders, and lifestyles. It is characterized by infrequent bowel movements, difficulty passing stools, and straining during bowel movements.

Constipation can be caused by a variety of factors, including inadequate fiber intake, insufficient fluid intake, lack of physical activity, certain medications, hormonal changes, and certain medical conditions.

In addition to these factors, pelvic floor dysfunction can also contribute to constipation. When the pelvic floor muscles are weak or tight, they can make it difficult for the bowels to move smoothly through the digestive tract. This can result in constipation, as well as other bowel disorders.

Symptoms of constipation can include infrequent bowel movements, hard stools, difficulty passing stools, abdominal pain and discomfort, and bloating. If constipation persists for an extended period of time, it can lead to more serious complications such as hemorrhoids, anal fissures, and rectal prolapse.

Treatment for constipation typically involves lifestyle modifications such as increasing fiber and fluid intake, increasing physical activity, and reducing stress. In some cases, laxatives or stool softeners may be prescribed to help alleviate symptoms.

Physical therapy is another treatment option for constipation caused by pelvic floor dysfunction. Pelvic floor physical therapy can help strengthen or relax the pelvic floor muscles, allowing for improved bowel function. Other treatments such as biofeedback, massage therapy, and acupuncture may also be effective in treating constipation.

If you are experiencing symptoms of constipation or other pelvic floor disorders, it is important to seek medical attention and speak with your healthcare provider about treatment options. With the right treatment and lifestyle modifications, you can improve your pelvic floor health and achieve better bowel function.

Other disorders

Pelvic floor dysfunction can also lead to other disorders such as interstitial cystitis, endometriosis, vulvodynia, and prostatitis. Interstitial cystitis is a chronic condition that causes bladder pain and frequent, urgent urination. Endometriosis is a condition where the tissue that normally lines the inside of the uterus grows outside of it, causing pain and inflammation. Vulvodynia is a chronic pain condition that affects the vulva, and prostatitis is a condition that causes inflammation and swelling of the prostate gland in men. These conditions can all be associated with pelvic floor dysfunction and can be improved with pelvic floor exercises and other treatments.

Chapter Eight

Causes of Pelvic Floor Disorders

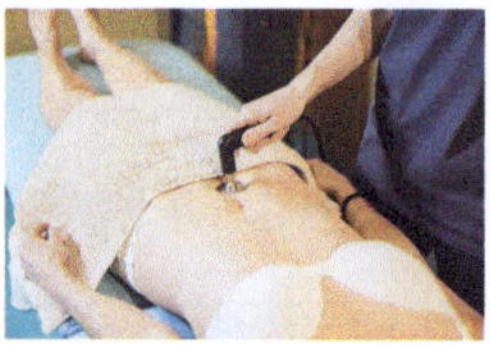

Pelvic floor disorders can have various causes, which can include:

1. Pregnancy and childbirth: The pelvic floor muscles and ligaments can be weakened or damaged during pregnancy and childbirth, particularly if there is a prolonged labor, a large baby or instrumental delivery.

2. Menopause: Hormonal changes during menopause can cause the tissues in the pelvic floor to weaken, leading to pelvic floor disorders.

3. Aging: As we age, the tissues in the pelvic floor can naturally lose their elasticity and strength, which can result in pelvic floor disorders.

4. Obesity: Carrying excess weight puts additional pressure on the pelvic floor, which can lead to pelvic floor disorders.

5. Chronic coughing: A persistent cough can cause the pelvic floor muscles to weaken over time, leading to pelvic floor disorders.

6. High-impact exercise: Participating in high-impact sports or exercises, such as running or jumping, can put strain on the pelvic floor and increase the risk of pelvic floor disorders.

7. Certain medical conditions: Certain medical conditions such as neurological disorders, connective tissue disorders and conditions that cause chronic coughing or constipation can also increase the risk of pelvic floor disorders.

8. Genetics: Some people may have a genetic predisposition to pelvic floor disorders.

It's important to note that while certain factors may increase the risk of pelvic floor disorders, anyone can develop a pelvic floor disorder.

Pregnancy and childbirth

Pregnancy and childbirth are among the most common causes of pelvic floor disorders. During pregnancy, the weight of the growing baby puts pressure on the pelvic floor muscles and can cause them to weaken. This can lead to problems such as urinary incontinence, pelvic organ prolapse, and pain during intercourse. Additionally, the process of giving birth can cause damage to the pelvic floor muscles, particularly if forceps or vacuum extraction is used.

The risk of pelvic floor disorders is higher for women who have had multiple vaginal deliveries, delivered a large baby, had a long or difficult labor, or had an episiotomy (a surgical cut made to widen the vaginal opening during delivery). Women who deliver via C-section are also at risk of pelvic floor disorders, as the procedure can weaken the pelvic floor muscles.

It's important for women to take care of their pelvic floor health during pregnancy and after giving birth. Prenatal exercise classes that focus on pelvic floor exercises, such as Kegels, can help strengthen the muscles and reduce the risk of developing a pelvic floor disorder. Women who experience symptoms of a pelvic floor disorder after giving birth should seek medical advice and treatment to prevent the condition from worsening.

Aging

As we age, the muscles and tissues in our body can weaken, including those in the pelvic floor. This can lead to pelvic floor disorders such as urinary incontinence and pelvic organ prolapse. Additionally, menopause in women can cause hormonal changes that affect the health of the pelvic floor muscles.

It's important to note that aging doesn't automatically mean you will experience pelvic floor disorders. Taking proactive steps to maintain the strength and health of the pelvic floor, such as doing exercises and maintaining a healthy lifestyle, can help prevent these issues.

Obesity

Obesity is a known risk factor for pelvic floor disorders. Excess weight puts pressure on the pelvic floor muscles and can weaken them over time. Studies have shown that women with a body mass index (BMI) of 30 or higher are at greater risk for urinary incontinence, pelvic organ prolapse, and other pelvic floor problems.

In addition to increasing the risk for pelvic floor disorders, obesity can also make it more difficult to treat these conditions. Weight loss can help to reduce symptoms and improve pelvic floor function, but it can be challenging for individuals with obesity to achieve and maintain a healthy weight.

It is important for individuals with obesity to seek treatment for pelvic floor disorders, as leaving these conditions untreated can lead to further complications and reduced quality of life. Treatment options may include pelvic floor exercises, behavioral changes, medication, or surgery, depending on the specific disorder and its severity.

Making lifestyle changes to achieve and maintain a healthy weight can also help to reduce the risk of developing pelvic floor disorders, as well as other health problems associated with obesity. A balanced diet, regular exercise, and support from healthcare professionals can all play a role in achieving this goal.

Menopause

Menopause can be a contributing factor in the development of pelvic floor disorders. As estrogen levels decrease during menopause, the tissues in the pelvic floor can become weaker and less flexible, leading to prolapse, urinary incontinence, and other related symptoms.

Additionally, menopause can cause changes in vaginal lubrication, making sexual intercourse painful and leading to a reduction in sexual activity, which can further contribute to weakening of the pelvic floor muscles.

Hormone replacement therapy (HRT) is often recommended to treat menopause symptoms, including pelvic floor disorders. However, the use of HRT can also have risks and should be discussed with a healthcare provider to determine the best treatment options for an individual.

Regular exercise, including pelvic floor exercises, can also help maintain pelvic floor health and prevent or alleviate symptoms related to menopause.

Hysterectomy

Hysterectomy is the surgical removal of the uterus. Depending on the type of hysterectomy performed, the cervix, ovaries, and fallopian tubes may also be removed. A hysterectomy can be performed for a variety of reasons, including pelvic pain, endometriosis, uterine fibroids, heavy or abnormal bleeding, and cancer.

Hysterectomy can lead to pelvic floor disorders because the removal of the uterus and other reproductive organs can weaken the pelvic floor muscles and connective tissues, leading to pelvic organ prolapse or urinary and fecal incontinence. Women who have had a hysterectomy may also experience a decrease in vaginal lubrication, which can cause pain during sexual intercourse. However, it is important to note that not all women who have had a hysterectomy will experience pelvic floor disorders, and many women can go on to have a healthy pelvic floor with proper care and exercise.

Chronic coughing

Chronic coughing is another cause of pelvic floor disorders. Coughing can put pressure on the pelvic floor muscles, causing them to weaken over time. This can lead to stress urinary incontinence or pelvic organ prolapse. People with chronic conditions such as asthma, bronchitis, or COPD are more likely to experience chronic coughing and are therefore at higher risk for developing pelvic floor disorders. Smoking can also lead to chronic coughing and increase the risk of pelvic floor disorders.

Heavy lifting

Heavy lifting is another cause of pelvic floor disorders. Repetitive heavy lifting, or even a single event of lifting something that is too heavy, can cause a strain on the pelvic floor muscles, leading to dysfunction. Jobs that require heavy lifting, such as construction work, may increase the risk of pelvic floor disorders. It is important to use proper lifting techniques to avoid putting unnecessary strain on the pelvic floor. This includes lifting with your legs, not your back, and avoiding twisting while lifting.

High-impact exercises

High-impact exercises such as running and jumping can also lead to pelvic floor disorders. The repeated pounding can cause the pelvic floor muscles to become weakened or damaged, leading to symptoms such as urinary incontinence and pelvic organ prolapse.

Additionally, certain types of exercises that place pressure on the pelvic floor, such as sit-ups, crunches, and weightlifting, can also contribute to the development of pelvic floor disorders.

It is important to maintain a balance between physical activity and pelvic floor health. Low-impact exercises such as yoga and swimming can help strengthen the pelvic floor without putting excessive strain on the muscles. It is also important to ensure proper technique and form during exercise to prevent damage to the pelvic floor.

Genetics

Pelvic floor disorders can also be caused by genetic factors. Studies have shown that there is a hereditary component to certain pelvic floor conditions, such as pelvic organ prolapse and urinary incontinence. If your mother or sister has had a pelvic floor disorder, you may be at higher risk of developing one as well. However, it is important to remember that genetic factors alone do not determine the development of pelvic floor disorders, and lifestyle factors also play a role.

Chapter Nine

Diagnosis of Pelvic Floor Disorders

Diagnosis of pelvic floor disorders begins with a physical examination and a detailed medical history. The medical professional may ask about the symptoms and their duration, as well as any relevant medical history. The next step may involve a pelvic exam, which involves an internal examination of the vagina and rectum. This may help the healthcare provider determine whether there is any damage or weakness in the pelvic floor muscles.

Further testing may be necessary to identify the underlying cause of the disorder. This may include urodynamic testing, where a healthcare provider may measure the strength and coordination of the bladder muscles. Other tests may include an ultrasound or MRI to assess the pelvic floor muscles and organs, and a colonoscopy to examine the rectum and colon.

It is important to note that pelvic floor disorders can often be misdiagnosed or underdiagnosed, as many individuals may be too embarrassed or uncomfortable to discuss their symptoms with their healthcare provider. It is important to seek medical attention if symptoms persist or interfere with daily life, as early intervention can lead to more successful treatment outcomes.

Pelvic exam

A pelvic exam is often the first step in diagnosing pelvic floor disorders. During the exam, the doctor will ask the patient to lie on their back with their feet in stirrups. The doctor will then visually examine the external genitalia for any signs of inflammation or irritation. They will also insert a speculum into the vagina to examine the cervix and check for any abnormalities.

The doctor may also perform a digital rectal exam, in which they insert a gloved finger into the rectum to check for any abnormalities in the pelvic area.

In some cases, the doctor may also order additional tests to help diagnose the specific type of pelvic floor disorder, such as urodynamic testing, imaging tests like an MRI or ultrasound, or a cystoscopy to examine the bladder.

Ultrasound

An ultrasound may be used to visualize the pelvic organs and muscles in motion to diagnose pelvic floor disorders. During this procedure, a handheld device (transducer) is placed on the abdomen or inserted into the vagina to create an image of the pelvic organs on a computer screen.

A pelvic ultrasound can be helpful in identifying structural abnormalities or organ prolapse. It can also provide information about bladder or kidney problems that could be contributing to urinary symptoms.

In addition to a pelvic ultrasound, doctors may also use other imaging tests such as MRI or CT scans to get a more detailed look at the pelvic area. These tests can help identify issues such as tumors, cysts, or abnormalities in the pelvic bones.

X-rays

X-rays are not a primary tool for diagnosing pelvic floor disorders, but they can be used to identify some underlying conditions such as pelvic bone fractures, tumors, or signs of arthritis. X-rays can also be used to monitor the position of certain devices or implants used to treat pelvic floor disorders. However, more advanced imaging methods such as MRI and CT scans are typically used to diagnose pelvic floor disorders.

MRI

Magnetic resonance imaging (MRI) is a non-invasive diagnostic imaging technique that uses a powerful magnetic field, radio waves, and a computer to produce detailed images of internal organs and tissues.

MRI can be useful in diagnosing pelvic floor disorders because it can provide highly detailed images of the pelvic region, allowing doctors to examine the muscles, ligaments, and other structures that make up the pelvic floor.

MRI can also help identify the extent of damage or prolapse in the pelvic floor muscles and assess any associated complications.

It is generally considered a safe and effective diagnostic tool, although some people with metal implants or other medical devices may not be able to have an MRI.

Urodynamics testing

Urodynamics testing is a series of tests that assess the functioning of the urinary tract. During this test, a thin, flexible tube with sensors is inserted into the bladder and the rectum or vagina. The bladder is filled with sterile water, and the sensors measure the pressure in the bladder and the urinary sphincter.

The tests performed during urodynamics testing include:

Cystometry: This measures how much urine the bladder can hold and how much pressure it generates when filling.

Pressure flow study: This measures the pressure in the bladder during urination.

Electromyography (EMG): This measures the electrical activity in the muscles of the pelvic floor and the sphincter.

Urethral pressure profile: This measures the pressure in the urethra during urination.

Urodynamics testing can provide information on the functioning of the bladder and the urethra, which can help in the diagnosis of pelvic floor disorders such as urinary incontinence and bladder dysfunction. The test is usually performed in a urology clinic or hospital by a specialist in urology or gynecology.

Chapter Ten

Treatment Options for Pelvic Floor Disorders

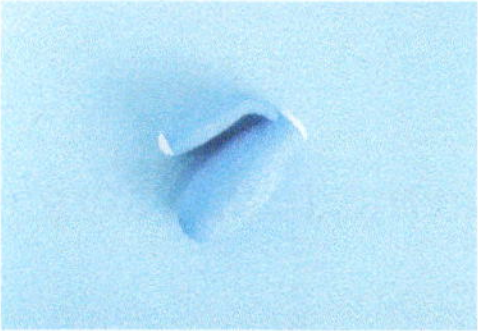

Treatment options for pelvic floor disorders depend on the specific disorder and its severity. Here are some common treatment options:

1. Pelvic floor muscle exercises: Kegel exercises are a type of pelvic floor exercise that can help to strengthen the pelvic floor muscles, improve bladder and bowel control, and reduce the risk of pelvic organ prolapse. Physical therapists can also help patients learn specific exercises to improve pelvic floor muscle function.

2. Medications: Medications such as antibiotics, anticholinergics, and alpha-blockers can help to treat urinary incontinence and other bladder problems.

3. Surgery: Surgery may be necessary for severe cases of pelvic organ prolapse or other pelvic floor disorders. There are different types of surgery available depending on the specific condition.

4. Biofeedback: Biofeedback is a technique that can help patients learn how to control and strengthen their pelvic floor muscles. A device is used to measure muscle activity and provide feedback to

the patient.

5. Vaginal pessary: A pessary is a device that is inserted into the vagina to support the pelvic organs and prevent pelvic organ prolapse.

6. Lifestyle changes: Making lifestyle changes such as losing weight, quitting smoking, and avoiding heavy lifting can help to improve symptoms of pelvic floor disorders.

7. Electrical stimulation: Electrical stimulation can be used to help strengthen the pelvic floor muscles and improve bladder and bowel control.

It is important to work with a healthcare provider to determine the best treatment options for your specific condition.

Pelvic floor exercises (Kegels)

Pelvic floor exercises, commonly referred to as Kegels, are often the first line of defense in treating pelvic floor disorders. These exercises aim to strengthen the muscles of the pelvic floor, improving their function and reducing the symptoms of incontinence, prolapse, and other disorders.

To perform Kegel exercises, you will need to locate the muscles of your pelvic floor. The easiest way to do this is to stop your urine stream mid-flow. The muscles you use to do this are your pelvic floor muscles.

To perform Kegels, squeeze your pelvic floor muscles as if you are trying to stop the flow of urine. Hold the contraction for five seconds, then release for five seconds. Repeat this cycle ten times in a row, several times a day.

In addition to traditional Kegels, there are other types of pelvic floor exercises that can be tailored to specific types of pelvic floor disorders. Your healthcare provider can recommend exercises specific to your condition.

It is important to note that it may take several weeks or even months of consistent exercise to see improvement in your symptoms. However, for many people, Kegels and other pelvic floor exercises can significantly reduce or eliminate the symptoms of pelvic floor disorders.

If you are unsure how to perform Kegels or other pelvic floor exercises, or if you have difficulty with them, speak with your healthcare provider or a pelvic floor physical therapist. They can help ensure you are performing the exercises correctly and tailor a plan specific to your needs.

Biofeedback

Biofeedback is a technique that involves the use of electronic devices to monitor and provide feedback about specific bodily functions, such as muscle activity. In the case of pelvic floor disorders, biofeedback can help patients learn to contract and relax the muscles in the pelvic floor correctly.

During a biofeedback session, sensors are attached to the skin over the muscles of the pelvic floor. The sensors send information to a monitor, which displays a graph or other visual representation of the muscle activity. Patients can then see how their muscles respond to different types of contractions and learn how to adjust their technique for optimal results.

Biofeedback is typically used in combination with pelvic floor exercises and can be helpful for patients who have difficulty identifying and contracting the correct muscles on their own. It may also be used to help patients overcome muscle imbalances or learn to coordinate the muscles of the pelvic floor with other muscles involved in urination and bowel movements.

Biofeedback is generally considered safe and non-invasive, although it may not be effective for all patients. The number and frequency of sessions required can vary depending on the severity of the pelvic floor disorder and the patient's response to treatment.

Electrical stimulation

Electrical stimulation is a treatment option that uses a mild electric current to stimulate the pelvic floor muscles. It can be used to treat both urinary and fecal incontinence, as well as pelvic pain. The electrical current is delivered through a small probe that is inserted into the vagina or rectum. The current causes the muscles to contract, which helps to strengthen them.

During the treatment, the patient may feel a tingling or mild electrical sensation in the area being treated. The intensity and duration of the treatment can be adjusted according to the patient's tolerance.

Electrical stimulation can be done in a healthcare provider's office or at home with a device that the patient can use themselves. The treatment may be recommended for a period of several weeks or months, depending on the severity of the condition.

As with any medical treatment, there may be side effects associated with electrical stimulation. These may include discomfort or pain during the treatment, skin irritation, or infection. It is important to discuss the risks and benefits of the treatment with a healthcare provider before starting.

Overall, electrical stimulation can be an effective treatment option for pelvic floor disorders, particularly when combined with other treatments such as pelvic floor exercises and lifestyle modifications.

Medications

There are several medications that can be used to treat pelvic floor disorders. Here are some common medications used:

Antimuscarinics: These medications are used to treat overactive bladder and urge incontinence. They work by relaxing the bladder muscles, reducing the urge to urinate.

Alpha-adrenergic agonists: These medications are used to treat stress incontinence. They work by tightening the muscles at the neck of the bladder, reducing urine leakage.

Hormone replacement therapy: This is used to treat menopausal symptoms, such as vaginal dryness, which can contribute to pelvic floor disorders.

Antibiotics: These are used to treat bacterial infections that can cause urinary tract infections and other pelvic infections.

Pain medications: These are used to manage pain associated with pelvic floor disorders, such as vulvodynia and pelvic pain syndrome.

Muscle relaxants: These medications are used to treat pain and discomfort associated with pelvic floor muscle tension.

It's important to consult with a healthcare provider before taking any medications, as they can have potential side effects and may not be appropriate for all individuals. In addition to medication, other treatment options for pelvic floor disorders may include physical therapy, surgery, and behavioral therapies.

Surgery

Surgery may be recommended in cases where non-invasive treatments have failed, or in more severe cases of pelvic floor disorders. The type of surgery will depend on the specific condition being treated.

For urinary incontinence, sling procedures may be performed, where a mesh is placed under the urethra to provide support. In cases of pelvic organ prolapse, surgery may involve the placement of a mesh or other supportive device to lift the pelvic organs back into place.

In severe cases of fecal incontinence, surgery may involve the repair or reconstruction of the anal sphincter. Pain during intercourse may be treated with surgery to repair tears or scar tissue in the pelvic floor muscles.

As with any surgery, there are potential risks and complications, such as infection, bleeding, and nerve damage. It is important to discuss the risks and benefits of surgery with your doctor before making a decision.

Recovery time after surgery will depend on the type of procedure and individual factors, such as age and overall health. It is important to follow your doctor's instructions for post-operative care, including rest and rehabilitation exercises to aid in recovery.

Chapter Eleven

Exercises to Strengthen the Pelvic Floor

Pelvic floor exercises, also known as Kegel exercises, can help strengthen the muscles in the pelvic area, which can help prevent or alleviate pelvic floor disorders. Kegel exercises involve contracting and relaxing the pelvic floor muscles, which support the bladder, bowel, and uterus. They are often recommended for women who are pregnant, have recently given birth, or are experiencing urinary or fecal incontinence. However, Kegel exercises can be beneficial for both men and women.

To do Kegel exercises, follow these steps:

Find the right muscles: To identify your pelvic floor muscles, try stopping the flow of urine when you are using the bathroom. The muscles you use to do this are your pelvic floor muscles.

Tighten the muscles: Once you have identified your pelvic floor muscles, contract them for 5-10 seconds. Make sure to breathe normally and not hold your breath.

Relax the muscles: After 5-10 seconds, release the contraction and relax the muscles for 5-10 seconds.

Repeat: Repeat the contraction and relaxation cycle 10-15 times, three times a day.

It may take several weeks or months of Kegel exercises before you start to see an improvement in your pelvic floor strength. It is important to continue doing the exercises, as they can help prevent pelvic floor disorders from worsening.

Variations of Kegel exercises may include using biofeedback, electrical stimulation, or weights to provide resistance during contractions, which can increase the effectiveness of the exercises. It is important to talk to your healthcare provider to determine which exercise routine is best for you.

Kegel exercises

Kegel exercises are one of the most well-known and effective exercises to strengthen the pelvic floor muscles. These exercises involve contracting and relaxing the pelvic floor muscles, which are the muscles that support the bladder, uterus, rectum, and small intestine.

To perform Kegel exercises, follow these steps:

Find the right muscles: To identify your pelvic floor muscles, try stopping the flow of urine midstream. If you can do this, you've found the right muscles. However, do not make a habit of doing this frequently, as it can lead to bladder problems.

Empty your bladder: Before you begin, empty your bladder to ensure that it is not full.

Tighten the muscles: Once you have found the correct muscles, tighten them and hold for three to five seconds. Be sure not to hold your breath or tighten your stomach, buttocks, or thigh muscles.

Relax the muscles: Release the muscles and relax for three to five seconds.

Repeat: Repeat the exercise 10 times, three times a day.

As you become more comfortable with Kegel exercises, you can gradually increase the duration of the contractions and the number of repetitions.

It is important to note that Kegel exercises may not be appropriate for everyone. If you have a pelvic floor disorder, it is recommended to consult a healthcare provider before starting any exercise regimen. They can provide guidance on the best exercises for your condition and make recommendations for the frequency and duration of your exercises.

Kegel

Balls

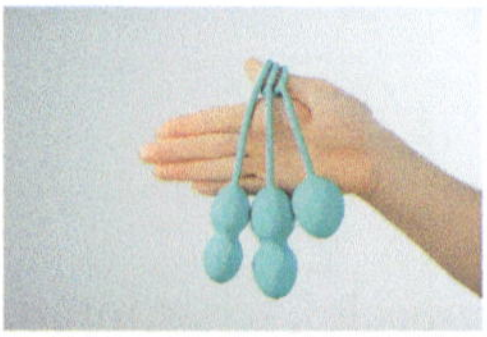

Kegel balls, also known as Ben Wa balls, are small, weighted balls that are designed to be inserted into the vagina to help strengthen the pelvic floor muscles. They come in a variety of shapes, sizes, and weights, and are typically made from materials like silicone or metal.

Using Kegel balls involves inserting the balls into the vagina and holding them in place by contracting the pelvic floor muscles. The weight of the balls creates resistance, which makes the exercises more challenging and effective.

Kegel balls are a popular choice for women looking to improve their pelvic floor health, as they are discreet, easy to use, and can be incorporated into daily routines. They are also often recommended by healthcare professionals as a non-invasive treatment for urinary incontinence and other pelvic floor disorders.

It is important to choose the right size and weight of Kegel balls for your individual needs, as using a ball that is too heavy or too large can cause discomfort or even damage to the pelvic floor muscles. It is also important to clean the balls thoroughly after each use to prevent the risk of infection.

Before starting any pelvic floor exercise routine, it is recommended to consult with a healthcare professional to ensure that the exercises are safe and appropriate for your individual needs.

Squats

Squats are a great exercise for the pelvic floor because they engage the gluteal muscles, which support the pelvic floor. Here's how to do a squat:

Stand with your feet shoulder-width apart and your toes pointing slightly outward.

Keeping your back straight, bend your knees and lower your body as if you were sitting down in a chair.

Stop when your thighs are parallel to the ground.

Push through your heels to stand back up.

It's important to keep good form when doing squats. Make sure your knees don't extend beyond your toes, and keep your weight on your heels. You can also try holding a weight or using resistance bands to increase the difficulty of the exercise.

Bridges

Bridges are another exercise that can help strengthen the pelvic floor muscles. To perform a bridge, lie on your back with your knees bent and feet flat on the floor. Slowly lift your hips up towards the ceiling, squeezing your glutes and pelvic floor muscles as you do so. Hold for a few seconds and then lower your hips back down to the floor. Repeat this exercise for several repetitions. Bridges also work the core and glutes, which can help support the pelvic floor muscles.

Lunges

Lunges are a great way to strengthen your pelvic floor muscles while also working your glutes and thighs. To perform a lunge:

Stand with your feet hip-width apart.

Take a large step forward with your right foot, keeping your left foot in place.

Bend your right knee and lower your body until your right thigh is parallel to the ground. Keep your left leg straight.

Push off with your right foot to return to standing.

Repeat on the other side.

To engage your pelvic floor muscles during lunges, focus on lifting them up and in as you lunge forward. You can also try doing mini pulses at the bottom of the lunge to really work those muscles. As you get stronger, you can hold weights in your hands to increase the difficulty of the exercise.

Planks

Planks are an effective exercise for strengthening the pelvic floor muscles, as well as the core and back muscles. Here's how to do a plank:

Begin on all fours with your hands shoulder-width apart and your knees hip-width apart.

Step your feet back, straightening your legs and coming into a high plank position.

Engage your core and hold the plank for 20-30 seconds.

Release and rest for 10-20 seconds.

Repeat the plank 3-4 times.

To make the plank easier, you can modify by dropping your knees to the floor or holding the plank for a shorter duration. To make the plank more challenging, you can try holding it for longer periods of time or adding movement, such as lifting one leg or arm off the ground.

Chapter Twelve

Diet and Lifestyle Changes for Pelvic Floor Health

The pelvic floor muscles play an important role in maintaining continence, supporting pelvic organs, and facilitating sexual function. To keep these muscles healthy, it is important to make certain diet and lifestyle changes.

One of the most important things you can do for your pelvic floor is to maintain a healthy weight. Being overweight or obese can increase the risk of pelvic floor disorders, including urinary incontinence and pelvic organ prolapse. Additionally, carrying extra weight can put extra strain on the pelvic floor muscles, leading to weakening over time.

Eating a healthy diet can also help maintain pelvic floor health. Eating foods high in fiber, such as fruits, vegetables, and whole grains, can help prevent constipation, which can put extra strain on the pelvic floor muscles. Drinking plenty of water is also important to keep stools soft and easy to pass.

Exercising regularly can also help keep the pelvic floor muscles strong. Cardiovascular exercise, such as walking or running, can improve circulation to the pelvic region, while strength training exercises can help build muscle in the pelvic floor and other areas. However, high-impact exercises like jumping or running can put extra strain on the pelvic floor, so it's important to balance these exercises with low-impact options, such as swimming or cycling.

Other lifestyle changes that can improve pelvic floor health include quitting smoking and avoiding heavy lifting, especially with poor lifting techniques. Proper lifting involves bending the knees and keeping the back straight, using the leg muscles to lift rather than the back muscles.

By making these diet and lifestyle changes, you can improve your pelvic floor health and reduce the risk of pelvic floor disorders.

Hydration

Drinking plenty of water is essential for overall health and can also help with pelvic floor health. Dehydration can cause constipation, which puts pressure on the pelvic floor and can contribute to pelvic organ prolapse and urinary incontinence. Aim to drink at least 8-10 glasses of water per day.

It is also important to avoid or limit diuretic beverages, such as coffee, tea, and alcohol, which can irritate the bladder and lead to increased urinary urgency and frequency.

Maintaining a healthy weight through a balanced diet and regular exercise can also improve pelvic floor health. Being overweight can put excess pressure on the pelvic floor muscles and lead to pelvic organ prolapse and urinary incontinence.

Finally, avoiding smoking can also help with pelvic floor health. Smoking can irritate the bladder and contribute to chronic coughing, which can strain the pelvic floor muscles.

High-fiber diet

A high-fiber diet is essential for maintaining healthy bowel movements and preventing constipation. Fiber helps to keep stool soft and bulky, making it easier to pass through the rectum and out of the body. A diet high in fiber can also help to reduce the risk of developing diverticulitis, a condition that can cause pain and inflammation in the colon.

Foods that are high in fiber include fruits, vegetables, whole grains, legumes, and nuts. Some examples of high-fiber foods include:

Apples, pears, and berries

- Broccoli, carrots, and kale
- Whole grain bread, pasta, and cereal
- Brown rice and quinoa
- Beans, lentils, and chickpeas
- Almonds, walnuts, and other nuts

In addition to eating a high-fiber diet, it is important to stay well-hydrated to maintain healthy bowel movements. Drinking plenty of water and other fluids can help to soften stool and make it easier to pass.

Maintaining a healthy weight through regular exercise and a balanced diet can also help to prevent pelvic floor disorders. Obesity and excess weight can put added pressure on the pelvic floor muscles, contributing to conditions such as urinary incontinence and pelvic organ prolapse.

Avoiding irritants (caffeine, alcohol, acidic foods)

Avoiding irritants such as caffeine, alcohol, and acidic foods is also important for pelvic floor health. These substances can irritate the bladder and bowels, causing them to become overactive and potentially contributing to incontinence or other pelvic floor disorders. It's a good idea to limit your intake of these substances or avoid them altogether if you notice that they worsen your symptoms.

In addition to avoiding irritants, maintaining a healthy weight is important for pelvic floor health. Being overweight or obese can put additional pressure on the pelvic floor muscles and increase the risk of developing pelvic floor disorders. Regular exercise can help with weight management and improve overall pelvic floor health, but it's important to avoid high-impact activities that can strain the pelvic floor muscles.

Finally, good bowel habits are also important for pelvic floor health. Straining during bowel movements can weaken the pelvic floor muscles and increase the risk of developing pelvic organ prolapse or other disorders. Maintaining regular bowel movements and using the correct technique for emptying the bowels can help prevent these issues.

Maintaining a healthy weight

Maintaining a healthy weight can also be helpful in promoting pelvic floor health. Being overweight can put excess pressure on the pelvic floor muscles, leading to weakness and dysfunction. Additionally, losing weight can reduce the risk of conditions such as pelvic organ prolapse and urinary incontinence. Eating a balanced diet and engaging in regular physical activity can help in achieving and maintaining a healthy weight.

It's important to note that weight loss should be achieved gradually, as rapid weight loss can also weaken the pelvic floor muscles. Working with a healthcare professional, such as a registered dietitian, can be helpful in developing a safe and effective weight loss plan that supports pelvic floor health.

Avoiding constipation

Constipation is one of the major causes of pelvic floor disorders, so it is important to avoid it by maintaining a healthy diet and lifestyle. Eating a diet that is high in fiber, drinking plenty of water, and getting regular exercise can all help prevent constipation. In addition, avoiding foods that are known to cause constipation, such as processed foods, dairy products, and red meat, can also be helpful.

If you do experience constipation, there are several things you can do to relieve it. Eating more fiber-rich foods, taking a fiber supplement, and drinking plenty of water can all help. In addition, regular exercise, especially exercises that work the abdominal muscles, can help stimulate the bowels and make it easier to pass stools. Finally, if you are still having trouble with constipation, your doctor may recommend a laxative or stool softener to help you go more easily.

Chapter Thirteen

Strategies for Coping with Pelvic Floor Disorders

Pelvic floor disorders can cause physical, emotional and social discomfort. However, it is possible to cope with these disorders and maintain a good quality of life. Here are some strategies that can help individuals cope with pelvic floor disorders.

Education: Education is the first and the most important step in coping with pelvic floor disorders. Understanding the disorder, the symptoms and the available treatments can help individuals take control of their health.

Pelvic floor muscle exercises: Regular pelvic floor muscle exercises, such as Kegels, can help strengthen the pelvic floor muscles, reduce the symptoms of pelvic floor disorders and improve quality of life.

Relaxation techniques: Relaxation techniques, such as deep breathing, meditation and yoga, can help reduce stress and anxiety, which can aggravate the symptoms of pelvic floor disorders.

Physical therapy: Physical therapy can help individuals with pelvic floor disorders to improve their physical function and quality of life. A physical therapist can design an exercise program tailored to the individual's specific needs.

Support groups: Joining a support group can help individuals cope with the emotional and social challenges of pelvic floor disorders. It provides a platform to share experiences, learn from others and find emotional support.

Behavioral therapy: Behavioral therapy can help individuals identify and change negative thought patterns and behaviors that aggravate the symptoms of pelvic floor disorders. It can also help individuals develop coping mechanisms to deal with the symptoms.

Medical treatments: In some cases, medical treatments such as medications, surgery or medical devices may be required to manage pelvic floor disorders. Consultation with a healthcare provider can help determine the most appropriate treatment.

Self-care: Engaging in self-care activities, such as taking a warm bath, getting a massage, or doing something enjoyable, can help reduce stress and promote relaxation.

Conclusion:

Coping with pelvic floor disorders requires a holistic approach that involves a combination of education, exercise, relaxation techniques, social support, medical treatment and self-care. The most important thing is to take control of your health, seek help when needed, and stay positive. With the right mindset and tools, it is possible to cope with pelvic floor disorders and lead a fulfilling life.

Pelvic floor physical therapy

Pelvic floor physical therapy is a specialized form of physical therapy designed to address pelvic floor disorders. This type of therapy is conducted by a specially trained physical therapist who has expertise in the musculoskeletal and neuromuscular structures of the pelvic region.

Pelvic floor physical therapy may involve exercises and techniques designed to help improve pelvic floor function, such as Kegels, biofeedback, and electrical stimulation. The therapist may also work with the patient to identify lifestyle factors that may be contributing to their pelvic floor disorder, such as poor posture or heavy lifting.

In addition to physical therapy, patients with pelvic floor disorders may benefit from other forms of treatment, such as medication or surgery. However, physical therapy is often considered an important first step in managing these conditions, as it can provide long-term relief and help prevent further damage to the pelvic floor muscles.

Support groups

Support groups can provide a valuable source of information and support for individuals experiencing pelvic floor disorders. These groups can help patients connect with others who are going through similar experiences, and provide a forum for discussing issues related to pelvic floor health.

Support groups may be in-person or online, and may be organized by healthcare providers, patient advocacy groups, or other organizations. They may offer educational resources, peer support, and opportunities to connect with healthcare professionals and other experts in the field.

In addition to support groups, many healthcare providers offer counseling or therapy to help patients cope with the emotional and psychological impact of pelvic floor disorders. This can include individual counseling, couples therapy, or other forms of support to help patients and their partners navigate the challenges of living with these conditions.

It's important to remember that living with a pelvic floor disorder can be challenging, and it's normal to experience a range of emotions, including frustration, anxiety, and depression. Seeking out support from others who understand what you're going through can be a valuable part of your treatment plan.

Mental health

counselling

Pelvic floor disorders can take a significant toll on a person's mental health. Chronic pain, discomfort, embarrassment, and lifestyle changes can lead to depression, anxiety, and other emotional struggles. Thus, it is crucial to address the mental health aspect of pelvic floor disorders and take steps to improve your well-being.

Here are some things to keep in mind:

Chapter Fourteen

What is the prognosis for Pelvic Floor Disorder

1. Seek Professional Help: Many people with pelvic floor disorders benefit from professional mental health counseling. A therapist can provide a safe space to discuss your emotions, provide coping strategies, and work with you to develop an action plan to improve your quality of life.

2. Practice Self-Care: Engage in activities that bring you joy, relaxation, and pleasure. This could include taking a warm bath, reading a book, or practicing mindfulness exercises.

3. Connect with Others: Joining a support group can help you feel less alone and provide a safe space to talk about your experiences with others who understand what you are going through. Social support can be an essential part of managing the emotional impact of pelvic floor disorders.

4. Practice Stress Management Techniques: Managing stress is an essential aspect of maintaining good mental health. Techniques such as deep breathing, meditation, or yoga can help you reduce your stress levels and improve your overall well-being.

5. Keep a Positive Outlook: Remember, many pelvic floor disorders are treatable, and most people experience significant improvements in their symptoms with proper care. It can be helpful to

keep a positive outlook and focus on the improvements you are experiencing rather than the challenges.

6. Don't Be Afraid to Ask for Help: Pelvic floor disorders can be complex and challenging to manage. Don't hesitate to ask for help from your healthcare provider, family, or friends. There is no need to suffer in silence, and support is available.

The prognosis for pelvic floor disorders varies depending on the specific disorder and individual circumstances. In general, however, many pelvic floor disorders can be managed with appropriate treatment and lifestyle changes. It is important to seek prompt medical attention if you are experiencing symptoms of a pelvic floor disorder, as early diagnosis and treatment can improve the chances of successful management. With the right interventions and ongoing care, many people are able to maintain good pelvic floor health and enjoy a good quality of life.

Coping with a Pelvic Floor Disorder

Living with a pelvic floor disorder can be challenging and uncomfortable, but there are several ways to cope with the condition and manage the symptoms. Here are some strategies for coping with a pelvic floor disorder:

1. Educate yourself: It is essential to learn as much as possible about your condition, including the causes, symptoms, and treatment options. Talk to your healthcare provider, read books and articles, and join support groups to learn more about your condition and connect with others who are going through the same experience.

2. Practice pelvic floor exercises: Pelvic floor exercises, such as Kegels, can help strengthen the pelvic floor muscles and improve symptoms such as urinary incontinence, pelvic pain, and pelvic organ

prolapse. Your healthcare provider or a pelvic floor physical therapist can guide you in performing these exercises correctly.

3. Maintain a healthy lifestyle: A healthy diet, regular exercise, and stress management can help manage pelvic floor disorder symptoms. Avoiding irritants such as caffeine, alcohol, and acidic foods can also help reduce symptoms.

4. Use supportive devices: Supportive devices such as pessaries, vaginal cones, and Kegel balls can help support the pelvic organs and improve symptoms of pelvic organ prolapse.

5. Seek professional help: Pelvic floor physical therapy, biofeedback, and medication can help alleviate symptoms of pelvic floor disorders. If necessary, surgery may be recommended.

6. Address emotional needs: Pelvic floor disorders can cause emotional distress and impact quality of life. Consider seeking mental health counseling or joining a support group to cope with the emotional impact of the condition.

7. Communicate with your healthcare provider: It is crucial to communicate openly with your healthcare provider about your symptoms, treatment options, and concerns. A collaborative approach between the patient and healthcare provider is essential in managing pelvic floor disorders.

Emotional impact of a Disorder Pelvic Floor

A Pelvic Floor Disorder can have a significant emotional impact on a person. Coping with the symptoms and impact of the disorder can be challenging and may lead to feelings of frustration, embarrassment, and anxiety. It is common for people to feel ashamed or self-conscious about the symptoms of a pelvic floor disorder, and it can be challenging to talk about these issues with others.

Living with a pelvic floor disorder can also affect a person's intimate relationships, as they may experience pain during sexual activity or feel uncomfortable discussing their symptoms with their partner. This can lead to feelings of isolation and a decreased quality of life.

It is essential for people living with a pelvic floor disorder to seek out support and resources to help them cope with their symptoms. This can include support groups, counseling, and therapy. With the right treatment and support, people with pelvic floor disorders can manage their symptoms and improve their overall quality of life.

Coping strategies for patients and caregivers

Coping with a pelvic floor disorder can be a difficult and stressful experience for patients and their caregivers. Here are some coping strategies that can help:

Seek support: Joining a support group can be a great way to connect with others who are going through the same experience. You can find support groups online or through your healthcare provider.

Take care of yourself: It is important to take care of your physical and emotional well-being. Eating a healthy diet, getting regular exercise, and practicing stress-reducing techniques like meditation or yoga can help.

Communicate with your healthcare provider: If you are experiencing discomfort or pain, or if you are feeling overwhelmed or anxious, be sure to talk to your healthcare provider. They may be able to offer additional treatment options or refer you to a mental health professional.

Educate yourself: Learning more about your condition can help you feel more in control and empowered. Talk to your healthcare provider, do research online, or attend educational events to learn more.

Be patient: Recovery from a pelvic floor disorder can take time. Be patient with yourself and trust in the treatment process. Celebrate small victories along the way and try to stay positive.

Chapter Fifteen

The role of diet in Pelvic Floor Disorders

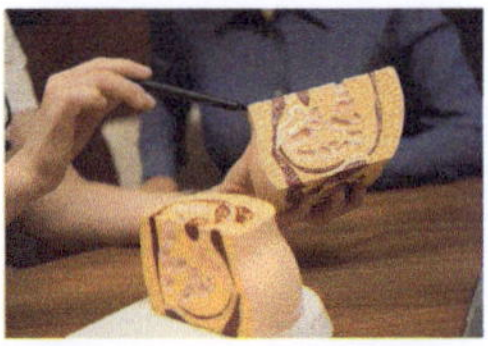

Maintaining a healthy diet can play a role in preventing or managing certain pelvic floor disorders. Here are some tips:

Stay hydrated: Drinking enough water is important to keep the body hydrated and maintain healthy bowel function.

Eat high-fiber foods: Fiber helps to prevent constipation and keeps bowel movements regular. Good sources of fiber include whole grains, fruits, vegetables, nuts, and seeds.

Limit caffeine and alcohol: Caffeine and alcohol can irritate the bladder and worsen symptoms of urinary incontinence.

Avoid spicy or acidic foods: Spicy or acidic foods can irritate the bladder and worsen symptoms of urinary incontinence.

Maintain a healthy weight: Being overweight or obese can put extra pressure on the pelvic floor muscles and worsen symptoms of pelvic organ prolapse.

Avoid constipation: Constipation can strain the pelvic floor muscles and worsen symptoms of pelvic organ prolapse and fecal incontinence. Eating a high-fiber diet, drinking enough water, and staying active can help prevent constipation.

Limit processed foods: Processed foods are often high in salt and sugar, which can contribute to inflammation and worsen symptoms of pelvic pain.

It's important to talk to a healthcare provider or registered dietitian for individualized advice on how to maintain a healthy diet and prevent or manage pelvic floor disorders.

Chapter Sixteen

The role of stress in Pelvic Floor Disorders

Stress can have a significant impact on pelvic floor health and can exacerbate symptoms of pelvic floor disorders. When a person is under stress, their body releases cortisol and other stress hormones, which can contribute to muscle tension and inflammation throughout the body, including in the pelvic floor.

Stress can also lead to poor habits that can contribute to pelvic floor disorders, such as poor posture, overeating, and neglecting exercise.

Learning how to manage stress can help improve pelvic floor health and reduce symptoms of pelvic floor disorders. This may involve practicing relaxation techniques such as deep breathing, meditation, or yoga, as well as incorporating regular exercise into a daily routine.

It is also important to address any underlying causes of stress, such as work or relationship issues, and to seek support from a therapist or counselor if necessary.

Chapter Seventeen

What are the risks and complications associated with a Pelvic Floor Disorder

Pelvic floor disorders can lead to a number of complications and health risks. For example:

1. Incontinence: Loss of bladder or bowel control can lead to social isolation, depression, and skin irritation.

2. Pain: Pelvic pain can lead to decreased sexual function, depression, anxiety, and decreased quality of life.

3. Prolapse: Pelvic organ prolapse can cause pain and discomfort, and in some cases, can require surgery.

4. Sexual dysfunction: Pelvic floor disorders can affect sexual function, leading to decreased sexual pleasure and difficulty achieving orgasm.

5. Constipation: Chronic constipation can lead to hemorrhoids, anal fissures, and other complications.

6. Infection: Some pelvic floor disorders, such as urinary incontinence, can increase the risk of urinary tract infections.

7. Interference with daily activities: Pelvic floor disorders can interfere with daily activities such as exercise, work, and travel.

It's important to seek treatment for pelvic floor disorders to prevent or minimize these complications and risks.

Chapter Eighteen

What happens if you don't fix your pelvic floor?

If you don't address and treat a weakened or dysfunctional pelvic floor, it can lead to a variety of complications and health issues. These can include urinary and/or fecal incontinence, pelvic organ prolapse, sexual dysfunction or pain, and chronic pain in the pelvic area. It can also lead to decreased quality of life, social isolation, and mental health issues such as anxiety and depression. In severe cases, surgery may be required to address pelvic floor disorders. It's important to seek medical attention and treatment as soon as possible to prevent further damage and improve overall pelvic floor health.

If you neglect to address your pelvic floor issues, it can lead to a range of negative consequences. Here are some of the possible outcomes of untreated pelvic floor disorders:

1. Incontinence: One of the most common symptoms of pelvic floor dysfunction is incontinence, which is the involuntary leakage of urine or feces. If left untreated, incontinence can become increasingly severe, leading to embarrassment, social isolation, and reduced quality of life.

2. Pelvic organ prolapse: Prolapse occurs when the pelvic organs (such as the bladder, uterus, or rectum) descend into the vaginal canal due to weakened pelvic floor muscles. If left untreated, pelvic organ prolapse can worsen, leading to severe discomfort

and difficulty with daily activities.

3. Sexual dysfunction: Pelvic floor dysfunction can cause sexual dysfunction, such as pain during intercourse, difficulty achieving orgasm, or decreased sexual desire. These symptoms can negatively impact romantic relationships and overall quality of life.

4. Chronic pain: Untreated pelvic floor dysfunction can lead to chronic pain in the pelvic area. This pain can be debilitating and make it difficult to perform daily activities or even sit for long periods.

5. Depression and anxiety: The physical symptoms associated with pelvic floor disorders can also lead to emotional distress, such as anxiety and depression. These conditions can further exacerbate physical symptoms and lead to a negative cycle of worsening symptoms.

6. Increased risk of other health problems: Pelvic floor disorders can increase the risk of other health problems, such as urinary tract infections, constipation, and sexual dysfunction. These issues can further complicate the management of pelvic floor dysfunction.

It is crucial to address pelvic floor issues as soon as they arise to avoid these negative consequences. Pelvic floor dysfunction is a treatable condition, and many effective treatment options are available. Seeking medical advice from a qualified healthcare professional can help identify the cause of your symptoms and develop an effective treatment plan.

Treatment options for pelvic floor disorders may include pelvic floor exercises, medication, or surgery, depending on the severity of the issue. Pelvic floor exercises, also known as Kegel exercises, can help strengthen the pelvic floor muscles and improve bladder and bowel control. Medications may be prescribed to help manage incontinence, while surgery may be necessary in severe cases of pelvic organ prolapse.

In addition to medical treatments, certain lifestyle changes can help manage pelvic floor issues. For example, maintaining a healthy weight, staying hydrated, and avoiding constipation can help reduce pressure on the pelvic floor muscles. Avoiding irritants such as caffeine and alcohol can also help manage symptoms of incontinence.

It is important to note that seeking treatment for pelvic floor disorders is not a sign of weakness. Pelvic floor dysfunction is a common issue that affects many people, and it is nothing to be ashamed of. Seeking help is the first step towards managing the condition and improving your overall quality of life.

Chapter Nineteen

Living with a Pelvic Floor Disorder

Living with a pelvic floor disorder can be challenging, but it's important to remember that there are many treatment options available that can help manage symptoms and improve quality of life. In addition to seeking medical treatment, there are lifestyle changes that can be made to help manage symptoms and improve pelvic floor health.

Some strategies for living with a pelvic floor disorder may include:

Practicing good pelvic floor hygiene: It's important to keep the pelvic area clean and dry to prevent irritation and infection. Wiping from front to back after using the toilet and avoiding harsh soaps or perfumes can help prevent irritation.

Avoiding activities that aggravate symptoms: Certain activities such as high-impact exercises, lifting heavy weights, or straining during bowel movements can aggravate symptoms of a pelvic floor disorder. Avoiding these activities or modifying them to reduce strain on the pelvic floor can help manage symptoms.

Using pelvic support devices: There are various devices available that can provide additional support to the pelvic floor, such as pessaries or support underwear. These devices can help manage symptoms and improve quality of life.

Maintaining a healthy lifestyle: Eating a balanced diet, staying hydrated, getting regular exercise, and reducing stress can help improve pelvic floor health and manage symptoms.

Seeking emotional support: Coping with a pelvic floor disorder can be emotionally challenging, and it's important to seek emotional support from friends, family, or a mental health professional.

Living with a pelvic floor disorder may require some adjustments, but with the right treatment and support, it is possible to manage symptoms and lead a fulfilling life.

Chapter Twenty

Quick tips

Maintaining a resilient pelvic floor is less about heroic gym sessions and more about weaving small, thoughtful habits into everyday life. Consider these practical ideas a menu—choose a few to start, revisit often, and add new ones as your confidence grows.

• Practice diaphragmatic breathing to let your pelvic floor relax and coordinate with your breath

• Schedule a daily "check-in" moment to gently contract and release the pelvic floor while seated

• Work with a certified pelvic floor physiotherapist for a personalized exercise plan

• Drink enough water to keep urine diluted and avoid bladder irritation

• Pause and fully empty your bladder rather than rushing restroom visits

• Adopt the "knuckles on knees" posture when sitting on the toilet to encourage easier bowel movements

• Incorporate fiber-rich foods such as oats, berries, and legumes to prevent constipation strain

- Use a small footstool to elevate your feet during bowel movements for better pelvic alignment

- Exhale as you lift heavy objects to reduce downward pressure on pelvic organs

- Swap high-impact workouts for low-impact options like swimming or cycling during recovery

- Strengthen your deep core muscles with slow, controlled abdominal drawing-in exercises

- Add side-lying leg lifts to tone hip stabilizers that support pelvic alignment

- Set reminders to stand and stretch every 45 minutes if you work at a desk

- Choose supportive footwear to maintain proper pelvic and spinal alignment

- Practice gentle yoga poses—child's pose, bridge, and happy baby—focused on breath awareness

- Try prenatal yoga classes during pregnancy to learn safe pelvic floor engagement

- Aim for a healthy body weight to minimize excessive load on pelvic tissues

- Wear breathable, cotton underwear to reduce moisture and irritation

- Limit caffeine and carbonated drinks if they trigger bladder urgency

• Keep a bladder diary for a week to identify fluid-intake patterns and leakage triggers

• Include omega-3-rich foods like salmon or flaxseed for anti-inflammatory benefits

• Use heat packs on the lower abdomen to soothe cramping pelvic muscles

• Experiment with perineal massage (with guidance) to increase tissue elasticity before birth

• Switch from tampons to menstrual cups or pads if internal pressure feels uncomfortable

• Do gentle pelvic tilts on all fours to mobilize the lower spine and pelvis

• Support your bump with a maternity belt in late pregnancy to offload the pelvic floor

• Rest with legs elevated on a pillow to reduce pelvic congestion at the end of the day

• Practice "sipping" breaths—quick inhales, slow exhales—to calm an overactive bladder

• Use a smartphone app to guide and track Kegel exercise routines

• Alternate between sitting and standing desks to vary pelvic loading

• Invest in a firm, supportive mattress to keep the spine neutral during sleep

• Place a pillow between your knees when side-sleeping to align hips and pelvis

• Limit prolonged coughing by treating seasonal allergies promptly

• Learn the "knack"—a timed pelvic floor contraction before sneezing or coughing

• Opt for squat-based strength moves with light weights instead of heavy barbell lifts

• Build upper-back strength with rows to counteract rounded posture that stresses the pelvic floor

• Choose whole grains over refined carbs to stabilize blood sugar and reduce inflammation

• Insert vaginal weights only under professional guidance to avoid overtraining

• Alternate hot and cold showers on the lower abdomen to boost circulation

• Massage the glutes and hip flexors with a foam roller to release surrounding tension

• Practice mindful relaxation techniques to lower chronic stress that can tighten pelvic muscles

• Add magnesium-rich foods like spinach and almonds to support muscle relaxation

• Replace sit-ups with modified forearm planks that engage the core without doming

• Squeeze a cushion between the knees during bridges to engage inner-thigh support

• Monitor medication side effects, such as constipation, that may affect pelvic function

• Choose high-rise, supportive leggings for workouts to gently hold the abdomen

• Use gentle, unscented soaps to avoid vulvar irritation

• Take short walks after meals to stimulate digestion and reduce bloating pressure

• Limit heavy lifting during the first six weeks postpartum unless cleared by your provider

• Try belly wrapping or compression garments post-delivery to support healing tissues

• Celebrate small gains—like one fewer night-time bathroom trip—to stay motivated

• Share your goals with a partner or friend for accountability and emotional support

• Join online forums or local groups focused on pelvic floor wellness for community tips

• Keep pelvic floor exercise equipment in plain sight as a visual reminder

• Set aside five minutes before bed for guided relaxation or meditation

• Use gentle perineal cooling pads after childbirth to ease swelling

• Adjust bike-seat height and tilt to avoid perineal pressure when cycling

• Adopt a staggered stance when standing for long periods to distribute weight

• Learn belly-laugh techniques that engage the diaphragm without straining the pelvic floor

• Tune into hunger and fullness cues to prevent overeating that increases abdominal pressure

• Train exhale during exertion (blowing out candles) to coordinate breath and pelvic support

• Seek assessment for diastasis recti if you notice abdominal doming during movement

• Use slow, controlled movements rather than momentum in resistance training

• Strengthen gluteal muscles with hip thrusts to support pelvic alignment

• Perform seated marches to gently engage core and pelvic stabilizers

• Explore Pilates sessions tailored to pelvic floor rehabilitation

• Replace prolonged sitting on soft couches with supportive chairs

• Keep stress-incontinence pads handy when starting new fitness routines

• Visualize the pelvic floor lifting like an elevator while inhaling to foster mind-muscle connection

• Experiment with biofeedback devices if you struggle to feel contractions

• Schedule regular check-ups with a urogynecologist for ongoing guidance

• Don't ignore persistent pelvic pain—seek professional evaluation promptly

• Use silicone-based lubricants to reduce friction during intimacy

• Practice gentle perineal stretching post-menopause under medical guidance

• Consider hormone therapy discussions if dryness contributes to discomfort

• Limit high-heeled shoes that tilt the pelvis forward and strain muscles

• Take brief deep-squat breaks (heels supported) to mobilize the pelvis

• Balance hip-flexor stretching with glute strengthening for optimal support

• Try water aerobics for buoyant, pelvic-friendly cardio

• Apply gradual progression—add only small increments of exercise intensity weekly

• Use hands-on cues (finger on perineum) to feel subtle pelvic movements during training

• Establish consistent sleep patterns to support tissue repair and hormone balance

• Add probiotic-rich foods like yogurt for gut health, aiding regular bowels

• Replace constipation-inducing iron supplements with slow-release forms if appropriate

• Start pelvic floor training during pregnancy's second trimester when energy returns

• Reduce refined sugar intake to lower systemic inflammation

• Shift coughing into the elbow crease to lessen downward abdominal force

• Use mindfulness body scans to detect unconscious pelvic tension

• Alternate front- and side-carrying positions when holding a baby

• Perform ankle pumps while sitting to improve circulation and reduce edema

- Wear compression socks on long flights to prevent pelvic congestion

- Guided imagery of waves lifting and dropping can enhance relaxation practice

- Keep a hand on the lower abdomen during Kegels to avoid bearing down

- Warm up with dynamic stretches before exercise to prep supportive muscles

- Reassess your progress monthly and tweak routines rather than pushing through plateau

- Seek counseling if pelvic issues affect body image or intimacy confidence

- Celebrate non-workout movement—gardening, housecleaning—as functional training

- Focus on quality over quantity in each pelvic floor contraction

- Practice gentle humming on the exhale to stimulate vagus-nerve relaxation

- Train balance with single-leg stands to enhance overall core stability

Chapter Twenty-One

Frequently Asked Questions.

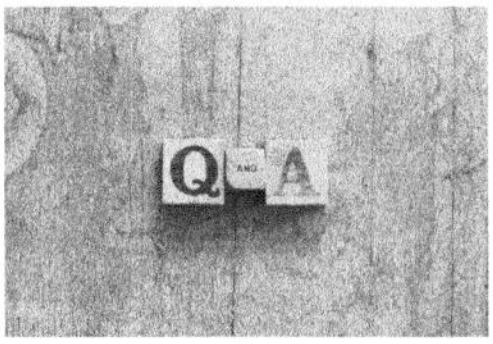

What causes a weak pelvic floor?

There are many different factors that can contribute to a weak pelvic floor. Some of the most common include: -Pregnancy and childbirth: The process of childbirth can cause the pelvic floor muscles to become stretched and even torn. This can lead to a loss of muscle tone and support, and can be a major cause of incontinence (leakage of urine or feces) after childbirth. -Aging: As we age, the muscles of the body can lose strength and tone. This includes the pelvic floor muscles. The loss of muscle tone in the pelvic floor can lead to incontinence and a feeling of heaviness or pressure in the pelvic region. - Obesity: Excess weight can put strain on the pelvic floor muscles and ligaments, leading to weakness and eventually, incontinence. - Chronic cough: If you suffer from a chronic cough, you may also be at risk for pelvic floor weakness. The frequent coughing can put strain on the muscles and ligaments of the pelvic floor, leading to weakness and incontinence. - Chronic constipation: chronic constipation can also lead to pelvic floor weakness. When you are constantly straining to have a bowel movement, the muscles and ligaments of the pelvic floor can become weak. This can eventually lead to incontinence.

If you are suffering from any of these problems, it is important to seek help. There are many different treatments available that can help to strengthen the pelvic floor muscles and reduce incontinence. These treatments can help you to regain control of your body and improve your quality of life.

How do you fix a weak pelvic floor?

The pelvic floor is a group of muscles that support the pelvic organs, including the bladder, uterus, and rectum. These muscles are located in the pelvis, and they attach to the pelvic bones and connect to the muscles of the pelvic floor. The pelvic floor muscles are responsible for keeping the organs in the pelvis in their proper place, and they also help to control the release of urine and feces. When the pelvic floor muscles are weak, they can no longer provide the same support to the organs, and they may also be unable to control the release of urine and feces. There are several ways to strengthen the pelvic floor muscles. One way is to do exercises that target these muscles. Kegel exercises, for example, are a type of exercise that can help to strengthen the pelvic floor muscles. Another way to strengthen the pelvic floor muscles is to use a device that provides electrical stimulation to the muscles. These devices are available without a prescription, and they can be used at home. If the pelvic floor muscles are very weak, surgery may be necessary to repair the muscles. This type of surgery is known as a pelvic floor reconstruction, and it can be performed by a urologist or a gynecologist. Pelvic floor reconstruction surgery is usually only recommended for women who have had a prolapse, or a hernia, of the pelvic organs. Surgery is not usually recommended for women who have weak pelvic floor muscles but no prolapse or hernia. The best way to prevent weak pelvic floor muscles is to avoid any activity that puts excessive pressure on the pelvic organs, such as lifting heavy objects, straining during bowel movements, or coughing excessively.

How do you know if your pelvic floor is strong?

It is important to have a strong pelvic floor in order to maintain bowel and bladder control, and to have a healthy sex life. There are a few ways to test whether or not your pelvic floor is strong. One way to test the strength of your pelvic floor is to try to stop the flow of urine when you are urinating. If you are able to do this, it is likely that your pelvic floor muscles are strong. Another way to test the strength of your pelvic floor is to insert a finger into your vagina and try to squeeze your pelvic floor muscles around it. If you are able to do this, again, it is likely that your pelvic floor muscles are strong. If you are not able to do either of these things, it may be that your pelvic floor muscles are weak. This is not necessarily a cause for concern, as there are a number of things that you can do to strengthen your pelvic floor. For example, you can do pelvic floor exercises (sometimes also called Kegel exercises). These exercises involve repeatedly contracting and relaxing the muscles of the pelvic floor. It is also important to be aware that the strength of your pelvic floor muscles can decline with age, so it is important to do exercises to keep them strong even if you have no currently observable problems. If you are post-menopausal, you may also experience a loss of pelvic floor muscle strength due to declining levels of estrogen. If you are concerned about the strength of your pelvic floor, or you are experiencing problems such as incontinence or pain during sex, it is important to talk to your doctor. They will be able to advise you on the best course of action.

How do I know if my pelvic floor is weak?

There are a few primary indicators of a weak pelvic floor. One frequent sign is the leakage of urine when coughing, laughing, or sneezing. This is called stress urinary incontinence, and is caused by a sudden increase in intra-abdominal pressure that weakens the muscles and tissues supporting the bladder. Other common symptoms include a feeling of heaviness or bulging in the vagina, difficulty starting or holding back the flow of urine, and difficulty passing stool or gas. These latter two problems are indicative of bowel or fecal incontinence, and are caused by a loss of rectal muscle tone. Childbirth is often cited as a leading cause of weak pelvic floor muscles, as the process of pushing a baby out can stretch and tear the muscles and supporting tissues. Other causes include being overweight or obese, chronic coughing, and chronic constipation. Age and menopause are also risk factors, as the hormonal changes of menopause can lead to the thinning and weakening of pelvic floor muscles. If you are experiencing any of these symptoms, it is important to consult with a healthcare professional to rule out other potential causes and to discuss treatment options. There are a number of different exercises and therapies that can help to strengthen the pelvic floor muscles and reduce or eliminate symptoms.

How can I tell if my pelvic floor is weak or tight?

There are a few different ways to tell if your pelvic floor is weak or tight. One way is to do a self-assessment. Another way is to ask your doctor or another healthcare provider to do an assessment. When you do a self-assessment, you can look for certain signs and symptoms that may indicate a weak pelvic floor. These signs and symptoms may include: leaking urine when you sneeze, cough, or laugh; leaking stool when you laugh, cough, or strain; pain in your pelvis or anus; pain during sex; and feeling like you need to constantly urinate or have a bowel movement. If you experience any of these signs or symptoms, it's important to see a doctor or other healthcare provider so they can properly assess your pelvic floor. There are a few tests that your doctor or another healthcare provider can do to assess your pelvic floor. These tests may include: a physical exam, during which your doctor or healthcare provider will feel for muscle tenderness, weakness, or tightness; an assessment of your posture and alignment; and a strength test, during which you will be asked to contract your pelvic floor muscles. Depending on the results of these tests, your doctor or healthcare provider will be able to determine if your pelvic floor is weak or tight. If your pelvic floor is weak, treatment may include exercises to strengthen the muscles. If your pelvic floor is tight, treatment may include stretching exercises to relieve the tightness. Regardless of the treatment, it's important to see a doctor or other healthcare provider so they can properly assess your pelvic floor and provide the most effective treatment.

How long does it take to strengthen pelvic floor?

When it comes to strengthening the pelvic floor, there is no one-size-fits-all answer. It depends on a number of factors, including how often you exercise, the intensity of your workouts, and your starting point. If you're starting from scratch, it's going to take longer to see results than if you're already in good shape. And if you can only commit to a few minutes a day, it's going to take longer than if you can block out an hour for a dedicated workout. That said, even if you can only spare a few minutes a day, you can still make progress. The key is to be consistent with your workouts and to gradually increase the intensity over time. If you commit to working out 3 times a week for 20 minutes at a moderate intensity, you can expect to see results in 4 to 8 weeks. If you up the ante to 4 or 5 times a week for 30 to 60 minutes at a higher intensity, you can expect to see results even sooner. Of course, how quickly you see results also depends on your goals. If you're just looking to improve your overall fitness, you might not need to exercise as intensely or as often as someone who's trying to rebuild muscle after an injury. The bottom line is that there's no magic number when it comes to strengthening your pelvic floor. It takes time and consistency to see results, but how long it takes ultimately depends on you and your goals.

Are squats good for pelvic floor?

In the modern world, it seems like there is an exercise or diet for everything. So, of course, the question arises: are squats good for the pelvic floor? The pelvic floor is a group of muscles that support the bladder, uterus, and rectum. They also help with sexual function and control urine flow. So, if these muscles are so important, does that mean we should all be doing squats to keep them healthy? There is no simple answer to this question. For some people, squats may help to strengthen the pelvic floor muscles and may even help to improve bladder control. However, for other people, squats may place too much pressure on the pelvic floor muscles and could actually lead to problems such as pelvic organ prolapse. If you are considering incorporating squats into your exercise routine to help improve your pelvic floor health, it is important to speak with your doctor or pelvic floor specialist first. They will be able to assess your individual situation and let you know if squats are right for you. Generally speaking, people with healthy pelvic floors should be able to perform moderate-intensity squats without any problems. If you have any kind of pelvic floor dysfunction, you may want to avoid squats or at least modify the way you do them. For example, if you have weak pelvic floor muscles, you may want to hold on to a sturdy chair or pole when performing squats. This will help to take some of the pressure off of your pelvic floor. If you do decide to squat, make sure that you are using proper form. This means keeping your feet hip-width apart and your back straight. You may also want to place your hands on your hips or extend them out in front of you for balance. When you squat down, breathe in and hold the position for a few seconds before slowly standing back up. If you experience any pain in your pelvic region during or after squats, it is important to stop and consult your doctor. While some discomfort is normal, pain is not. If you continue to experience pain, it could be a sign of an underlying condition and you may need to seek medical help. Overall, there is no definitive answer to whether or not squats are good for the pelvic floor. It really depends on the individual and their unique situation. If you have any concerns, be sure to speak with your doctor before trying squats or any other new exercise.

It's important for everyone to know about the pelvic floor, especially people with a vagina. The pelvic floor is a group of muscles and ligaments that support the pelvic organs and control the opening and closing of the urethra and anal canal. When these muscles are weak, it can lead to problems like incontinence and prolapse. Strengthening the pelvic floor muscles can help to prevent these problems.

How does a physio check pelvic floor?

A physiotherapist will check your pelvic floor by doing an internal examination. This involves putting a gloved finger into your vagina or rectum. The therapist will feel for any bulges or weak spots in the pelvic floor muscles. They will also assess your muscle tone and coordination. This examination can be done standing, sitting, or lying down. It is important to relax the muscles of your pelvic floor during the examination. Otherwise, the therapist will not be able to accurately assess the condition of your pelvic floor. After the internal examination, the physiotherapist will likely want to see you perform a series of exercises. This will help to further assess your muscle function. The therapist may also give you instructions on how to perform these exercises at home. The physiotherapist will use all of this information to develop a treatment plan specifically for you. This plan may include exercises, lifestyle changes, and other interventions. The goal of treatment is to improve the function of your pelvic floor muscles and reduce your symptoms.

Is it too late to fix my pelvic floor?

It is estimated that one in three women will experience some form of Pelvic Floor Dysfunction (PFD) in their lifetime. PFD can lead to a number of problems including incontinence, prolapse, pelvic pain, and sexual dysfunction. The good news is that it is never too late to fix your pelvic floor. There are a number of treatments available, both surgical and non-surgical, that can help to improve your symptoms. If you are suffering from PFD, the first step is to consult with a pelvic floor specialist. They will be able to assess your individual case and recommend the best course of treatment. In some cases, pelvic floor physical therapy may be recommended. This involves doing specific exercises and stretches to strengthen the muscles of the pelvic floor. If physical therapy is not effective, or if your symptoms are severe, you may be a candidate for surgery. There are a number of different surgical procedures that can be used to treat PFD. The type of surgery that is right for you will depend on the severity of your symptoms and the underlying cause of your PFD. For example, if you are suffering from incontinence, you may be a candidate for a sling procedure, which involves placing a support around the urethra to help prevent leakage. If you are suffering from prolapse, you may be a candidate for a sacral colpopexy, which involves attaching the prolapsed organ (usually the uterus) back to the sacrum. No matter what treatment option you and your pelvic floor specialist decide on, it is important to remember that it is never too late to fix your pelvic floor. With the right treatment, you can improve your symptoms and live a normal, healthy life.

How many times a day should you do pelvic floor?

Pelvic floor exercises, also commonly known as Kegel exercises, are a vital part of maintaining pelvic floor health. So how many times a day should you do pelvic floor exercises? The simple answer is: as often as you can! Ideally, you should be aiming to do at least 3 sets of pelvic floor exercises every day. Each set should consist of 10-15 repetitions. And don't worry if you can't do the full 15 repetitions to start with – just do as many as you can and build up gradually. Remember, the key to doing pelvic floor exercises effectively is to focus on the muscles themselves, not on the movement. So, even if you're just sitting at your desk or lying in bed, you can still do a few quick sets of pelvic floor exercises. There are a few different ways to do pelvic floor exercises, so experiment and find the method that works best for you. For example, you can try: - Squeezing and lifting your pelvic floor muscles as if you're trying to stop yourself from passing wind or urine. - Pretending to hold in a bowel movement and then letting go. - Tensing the muscles around your back passage as if you're trying to avoid passing stool. - Draw your pelvic floor muscles up and in, as if you're trying to lift your pubic bone. The most important thing is that you focus on the muscles themselves and not on the movement. So, even if you're just sitting at your desk or lying in bed, you can still do a few quick sets of pelvic floor exercises. If you're not sure whether you're doing the exercises correctly, don't worry – there are plenty of resources available to help you, including apps, DVDs, and books. You can also ask your GP or a Continence and Women's Health Physiotherapist for advice.

How should I sit to strengthen my pelvic floor?

Sitting is often thought of as a restful position, but did you know that how you sit can actually have an effect on your pelvic floor? The pelvic floor is a group of muscles and tissue that supports the bladder, uterus, and rectum, and helps control urinary and bowel movements. If these muscles are weak, it can lead to problems like incontinence or prolapse. Here are a few tips on how to sit in a way that will help strengthen your pelvic floor: -Sit up straight with your shoulders back and your head up. This may not be the most comfortable position at first, but it will help you use your core muscles and engage your pelvic floor. -Avoid crossing your legs. This can put extra pressure on your pelvic floor and can lead to urinary leakage.

-Try not to slouch. This puts pressure on your pelvic floor and can lead to prolapse or incontinence. -When getting up from a chair, do not round your back. Instead, use your leg muscles to stand up straight. This will help to avoid putting unnecessary pressure on your pelvic floor.

What activities strengthen pelvic floor?

The pelvic floor is a group of muscles and ligaments that form a bowl-shaped floor at the base of the pelvis. The pelvic floor supports the pelvic organs, including the bladder, uterus, and rectum. There are many different muscles and ligaments that make up the pelvic floor, and these muscles can be divided into two main groups: the levator ani muscles and the coccygeus muscle. The levator ani muscles are a group of three muscles that originate from the pelvis and attach to the ischium (the lower part of the hip bone). These muscles are the iliococcygeus, pubococcygeus, and puborectalis. The levator ani muscles support the pelvic organs and help to keep them in place. The coccygeus muscle is a triangular muscle that attaches to the sacrum (the triangular bone at the base of the spine) and the coccyx (the tailbone). The coccygeus muscle supports the pelvic floor and helps to keep the pelvic organs in place. There are many different activities that can help to strengthen the pelvic floor. These activities include: - Kegel exercises: Kegel exercises are a type of exercise that helps to strengthen the pelvic floor muscles. To do a Kegel exercise, tighten the muscles of the pelvic floor as if you are trying to stop urinating. Hold this contraction for 10 seconds, and then relax for 10 seconds. Repeat this 10 times. - Pelvic floor muscle contractions: Pelvic floor muscle contractions are another type of exercise that helps to strengthen the pelvic floor muscles. To do a pelvic floor muscle contraction, tighten the muscles of the pelvic floor as if you are trying to stop urinating. Hold this contraction for 5 seconds, and then relax for 5 seconds. Repeat this 10 times. - Bridging: Bridging is an exercise that helps to strengthen the muscles of the lower back and the pelvic floor. To do a bridge, lie on your back with your knees bent and your feet flat on the floor. Raise your hips off the floor, and hold this position for 10 seconds. Repeat this 10 times. - Squats: Squats are an exercise that help to strengthen the muscles of the legs and the pelvic floor. To do a squat, stand with your feet shoulder-width apart and your hands at your sides. Lower your body down as if you are going to sit in a chair. Stop when your thighs are parallel to the floor, and then stand back up. Repeat this 10 times. These are just some of the many different activities that can help to strengthen the pelvic floor. Remember, it is important to talk to your doctor before starting any new exercise routine.

How can I strengthen my pelvic floor without kegels?

The pelvic floor is a group of muscles and ligaments that forms a bowl-shaped sling at the base of the pelvis. These muscles and ligaments support the organs in the pelvis, including the bladder, uterus, and rectum. The pelvic floor muscles also help to control the flow of urine and feces. Kegel exercises are often recommended as a way to strengthen the pelvic floor muscles. However, there are other ways to strengthen these muscles without doing kegels. One way to strengthen the pelvic floor muscles is to practice Pilates. Pilates is a form of exercise that emphasizes the control of the body through the core muscles. The pelvic floor muscles are part of the core muscles, so by doing Pilates exercises, you can help to strengthen these muscles. Another way to strengthen the pelvic floor muscles is to do yoga. Yoga is an ancient form of exercise that helps to improve flexibility and muscle strength. There are many different yoga poses that can help to strengthen the pelvic floor muscles. If you are pregnant, you can also help to strengthen your pelvic floor muscles by doing perineal massage. Perineal massage is a type of massage that is done to the perineum, which is the area between the vagina and the anus. This type of massage can help to improve the elasticity of the pelvic floor muscles, which can make them stronger.

No matter which method you choose to help strengthen your pelvic floor muscles, it is important to be consistent with your exercises. Doing pelvic floor exercises on a regular basis can help to improve your overall health and well-being.

What does a prolapse feel like inside?

A prolapse is when one or more of your pelvic organs drop down from their normal position and press against the wall of your vagina. prolapses can be very uncomfortable. They can cause a sense of fullness or pressure in your pelvis, pain during sex, pain when you urinate or have a bowel movement, and difficulty urinating or having a bowel movement. Some women also have incontinence (leaking urine) or constipation. Most prolapses are not painful, but some can be. It depends on the size of the prolapse and where it is pressing on your vagina. If the prolapse is small, you may not feel anything at all. If the prolapse is larger, it can press on the nerves in your pelvis and cause pain. There are many different types of prolapse, and they can all feel different. The most common type of prolapse is uterine prolapse, which can cause a feeling of pressure or fullness in your pelvis. It may also cause pain during sex, and you may feel like your uterus is going to fall out of your vagina. uterine prolapse can also cause difficulty urinating or having a bowel movement, and you may leak urine when you cough or sneeze. Other types of prolapse include vaginal prolapse, which can cause a feeling of pressure or fullness in your pelvis, and rectal prolapse, which can cause a feeling of fullness or pressure in your anus. If you have a prolapse, it is important to see your doctor so that they can diagnose the type of prolapse and determine the best treatment for you. Treatment for prolapse typically includes pelvic floor exercises and surgery.

The pelvic floor is an essential part of the human body, and its importance should not be underestimated. It supports the organs in the pelvis and helps to keep them in place, as well as playing a role in sexual function and urination. This means that any problems with the pelvic floor can have a significant impact on a person's quality of life. Fortunately, there are treatments available for pelvic floor disorders, and with the help of a qualified healthcare professional, most people can find relief. With proper care and management, the pelvic floor can remain healthy and functional for a lifetime.

Is it normal to pee every 2 hours?

According to the National Association for Continence, about 25 million Americans experience urinary incontinence (UI) - the involuntary leakage of urine. While UI can happen to anyone, women are particularly prone to this condition due to pregnancy, childbirth, and menopause. UI can be a real nuisance, affecting your quality of life and causing you to feel embarrassed and frustrated. One of the most common questions women with UI ask is whether or not their frequency of urination is normal. Here's the thing: there is no "normal" when it comes to how often you should urinate. This varies from person to person, and is largely dependent on how much fluid you take in throughout the day. If you're drinking a lot of water or other fluids, you'll likely need to urinate more frequently. On the other hand, if you're not drinking enough fluids, you may urinate less often. There are, however, some general guidelines you can follow. The average person urinates between 6 and 8 times a day. If you're urinating more than 8 times a day, it's considered frequent urination. And if you're urinating more than 10 times a day, it's considered excessive urination. Excessive urination can be a sign of an underlying medical condition, such as diabetes or a urinary tract infection. If you're urinating frequently and it's causing you distress, it's best to see a doctor to rule out any potential health issues. Incontinence can also cause frequent urination. If you're leaking urine when you cough, sneeze, or laugh, it's likely that you have UI.

UI can be treated with medication, pelvic floor muscle exercises, or surgery. So, to answer the question, is it normal to pee every 2 hours? It depends. If you're drinking a lot of fluids, it's perfectly normal. But if you're not drinking enough fluids or you're leaking urine, it's best to see a doctor.

Does sitting on the toilet weaken pelvic floor muscles?

When it comes to our health, we often take for granted the simple act of using the restroom. However, there is more to consider than just proper hygiene when using the toilet. For example, did you know that sitting on the toilet can actually weaken your pelvic floor muscles? The pelvic floor is a hammock-like muscle that stretches from the pubic bone to the tailbone, and acts as a support for the bladder, intestines, and uterus. Like any muscle in our body, the pelvic floor can become weak from disuse. And since we typically use only our leg muscles when sitting on the toilet, the pelvic floor doesn't get the same workout. So, does that mean we should all switch to squatting on the toilet? Well, not necessarily. While some experts believe that squatting is the ideal position for using the restroom, others say that it's more important to focus on strengthening the pelvic floor muscles with exercises like Kegels. The bottom line is that if you're concerned about weakening your pelvic floor muscles, the best thing you can do is to pay attention to your body and be aware of your bathroom habits. And if you're ever in doubt, consult with a medical professional.

Do pelvic floor exercises make you poop?

A lot of people think that doing pelvic floor exercises will make them poop. But the truth is, there is no scientific evidence to support that claim. The pelvic floor is a group of muscles that support the pelvis and help to control bowel movements. So, when you do pelvic floor exercises, you are strengthening these muscles. There are many different reasons why people might think that doing pelvic floor exercises will make them poop. One reason is that they think the exercises will put pressure on the rectum and cause a bowel movement. Another reason is that they think the exercises will stimulate the nerves that control the bowel movement. However, there is no scientific evidence to support these claims. In fact, there is no evidence that doing pelvic floor exercises will make you poop. If you are concerned about your bowel movements, or if you are having trouble controlling your bowel movements, you should talk to your doctor. They can help you find the cause of the problem and recommend the best treatment.

What should I expect at my first pelvic floor physio?

There are a number of things that you can expect when you go to your first pelvic floor physio appointment. Your physio will likely ask you about your medical history and any symptoms that you are currently experiencing. They may also perform a physical examination, which may include an internal examination. Your physio will then develop a treatment plan specifically for you. This may involve a range of different techniques, such as pelvic floor muscle exercises, electrical stimulation, and advice on lifestyle changes. You can expect to see a significant improvement in your symptoms after a few sessions of pelvic floor physio.

How painful is pelvic floor therapy?

How painful is pelvic floor therapy? There are different types of pelvic floor therapy, and the pain level can vary depending on the individual and the specific therapy being used. Some people may experience little to no pain during therapy, while others may feel some discomfort. Trigger point release therapy is one type of pelvic floor therapy that may cause some pain. This type of therapy involves the release of tight muscles in the pelvic floor. The therapist will apply pressure to specific areas in the muscle to release the tension. This can cause some discomfort, but should not be overly painful. Another type of pelvic floor therapy is myofascial release therapy. This type of therapy involves stretching and massaging the connective tissue in the pelvic floor. This can also cause some discomfort, but should not be overly painful. Pelvic floor therapy can also be done using electrical stimulation. This type of therapy uses electrical currents to help relax the muscles in the pelvic floor. This can cause some discomfort, but is generally not painful. Overall, pelvic floor therapy is not typically painful. However, some people may experience some discomfort during therapy. If the discomfort is severe, the therapist can adjust the therapy to make it more comfortable.

Is pelvic floor physio worth it?

There is no one-size-fits-all answer to this question, as the benefits of pelvic floor physiotherapy will vary depending on the individual's specific situation. However, in general, pelvic floor physiotherapy can be an extremely effective treatment for a wide range of problems, including urinary incontinence, pelvic pain, and sexual dysfunction. For many people, the most significant benefit of pelvic floor physiotherapy is the improvement in urinary incontinence. Urinary incontinence is a very common problem, particularly for women, and can be very debilitating. Pelvic floor physiotherapy can help to strengthen the muscles that support the bladder, making it less likely for urine to leak out. Pelvic floor physiotherapy can also be helpful for treating pelvic pain. Pelvic pain can be caused by a number of different things, including muscle tightness, trigger points, and scar tissue. Pelvic floor physiotherapy can help to release muscle tightness and trigger points, as well as break down scar tissue. Sexual dysfunction is another common problem that can be helped by pelvic floor physiotherapy. Pelvic floor physiotherapy can help to release muscle tightness and trigger points, as well as improve blood flow to the area. This can lead to improved sexual function and satisfaction. Overall, pelvic floor physiotherapy can be an extremely effective treatment for a wide variety of problems. If you are experiencing any of the problems mentioned above, pelvic floor physiotherapy may be worth considering.

Can you strengthen your pelvic floor after 50?

Around 50 years old, many women start to experience changes in their bodies. Their skin becomes drier and thinner, they may start to feel aches and pains more often, and they may notice changes in their sexual health. One common change is a weakening of the pelvic floor muscles. The pelvic floor muscles support the bladder, uterus, and rectum. They also help with sexual function. When these muscles are weak, it can lead to problems like urinary incontinence, prolapse (when organs fall out of place), and sexual dysfunction. So, can you strengthen your pelvic floor after 50? The short answer is yes! Just like any other muscle in your body, the pelvic floor muscles can be strengthened with exercise. Kegel exercises are the most common pelvic floor exercises. To do a Kegel, simply squeeze the muscles you would use to stop the flow of urine. Hold the squeeze for three to five seconds, then relax for three to five seconds. Repeat 10 to 20 times. If you're not sure you're doing a Kegel correctly, you can ask your doctor or pelvic floor physical therapist to check. Pelvic floor exercises can be done anywhere, at any time. You can do them while you're sitting at your desk, or watching TV. You don't need any equipment, and no one else needs to know you're doing them. Start slowly, with just a few reps a day. As your muscles get stronger, you can add more reps, or hold the squeeze for longer. In addition to Kegel exercises, there are other things you can do to strengthen your pelvic floor. Regular aerobic exercise can help, as can weightlifting and Pilates. Avoiding constipation is also important, as straining to have a bowel movement can weaken the pelvic floor muscles. If you're experiencing urinary incontinence, prolapse, or sexual dysfunction, talk to your doctor. He or she can help you determine if the cause is a weak pelvic floor, and if so, recommend exercises to help strengthen the muscles.

The pelvic floor is a group of muscles, ligaments, and connective tissues that support the pelvic organs, including the bladder, uterus, and rectum. The pelvic floor muscles also aid in urinary and bowel control. While the pelvic floor is often associated with pregnancy and childbirth, it plays an important role in the health of all women.

What organs form the pelvic diaphragm?

The pelvic floor is a complex system of muscles, ligaments, and connective tissues that forms the base of the pelvis. This system supports the pelvic organs and the weight of the body above it. The pelvic diaphragm is a muscular sheet that separates the pelvis from the abdomen. It is made up of three main components: the pubococcygeus, the iliococcygeus, and the puborectalis. The pubococcygeus muscle is a triangular muscle that attaches to the pubic bone in the front and the tailbone in the back. This muscle forms the major part of the pelvic floor and is responsible for urinary continence and sexual function. The iliococcygeus muscle is a sheet of muscle that runs along the sides of the pelvis. It attaches to the lower part of the pelvis and helps to support the organs. The puborectalis muscle is a small muscle that Forms a sling around the rectum. This muscle helps to control bowel movements. The pelvic floor muscles work together to support the pelvic organs and the body above it. these muscles also work to control bowel movements and urination. The pelvic floor muscles are important for sexual function and for providing control during intercourse.

What is the difference between diaphragm and pelvic diaphragm?

The human diaphragm is a muscular and fibrous membrane that separates the thoracic cavity from the abdominal cavity. The diaphragm acts as a muscle of respiration, meaning it contracts and relaxes to help with the inhalation and exhalation of air. The pelvic diaphragm is a similar muscular and fibrous structure, but it is located between the pelvis and the perineum. The pelvic diaphragm acts as a muscle of urination and defecation, meaning it contracts and relaxes to help with the elimination of waste from the body. While both the diaphragm and the pelvic diaphragm are muscular and fibrous structures that help to separate the Thoracic and abdominal cavities, respectively, the main difference between the two is their function. The diaphragm acts as a muscle of respiration while the pelvic diaphragm acts as a muscle of urination and defecation. Both muscles are necessary for the proper function of the respective systems, but the diaphragm is responsible for the inhalation and exhalation of air and the pelvic diaphragm is responsible for the elimination of waste from the body.

What are the two parts of the pelvic diaphragm?

The pelvic diaphragm is a sheet of muscle and connective tissue that extends across the pelvis. It is divided into two parts: the levator ani and the coccygeus. The levator ani is a group of muscles located in the pelvis that support the pelvic organs and help to close the pelvic outlet. The levator ani consists of the pubococcygeus, the iliococcygeus, and the puborectalis. The coccygeus is a muscle that is located at the base of the spine. It attaches to the sacrum and the coccyx, and stabilizes the pelvis.

How do you release the pelvic diaphragm?

Your pelvic floor is a hammock of muscles, ligaments and connective tissue that supports your bladder, uterus and rectum. It stretches from your pubic bone in the front, to your tailbone in the back. The pelvic floor muscles are important for two main reasons. First, they help to control the flow of urine, so that you can "hold it" when you need to. Second, they are a key player in sexual function, providing the necessary support for sexual organs and aiding in orgasm. So how do you release the pelvic diaphragm? Unfortunately, there is no one-size-fits-all answer to this question. Each person's pelvic floor is unique, so what works for one person may not work for another. However, there are some general tips that can help. One of the best things you can do is to find a good pelvic floor physiotherapist. A physio will be able to assess your individual needs and create a tailored exercises program that is right for you. Kegel exercises are also a great way to strengthen and tone the pelvic floor muscles. Once these muscles are stronger, they will be better able to support your organs and control urinary flow. Regular aerobic exercise and stretching can also help to improve the flexibility and strength of the pelvic floor muscles. If you are struggling to release your pelvic diaphragm on your own, there are some medical devices that can help. Vaginal dilators are one option that can be prescribed by a doctor or pelvic floor physiotherapist. Dilators come in different sizes and are used to gradually stretch the pelvic floor muscles. This allows them to better support the organs and improve urinary control. Another option is electrical stimulation, which uses electrical currents to stimulate the pelvic floor muscles. This can be done externally, through the skin, or internally, through a vaginal or anal probe. Electrical stimulation has been shown to be effective in treating urinary incontinence and can also help to improve sexual function. If you are struggling to release your pelvic floor muscles, there are many options available to you. Finding the right one will depend on your individual needs and preferences. However, with the help of a pelvic floor physiotherapist or doctor, you should be able to find a treatment that works for you and helps you to regain control of your pelvic floor.

Does walking strengthen pelvic floor muscles?

It is a common belief that walking or any other kind of movement strengthens the pelvic floor muscles. However, there is no scientific evidence to support this belief. The pelvic floor muscles are actually not very active during walking or other movements. They are mainly used to keep the urinary and anal sphincters closed and to support the pelvic organs. The pelvic floor muscles can be strengthened through specific exercises, but walking is not one of them. Kegel exercises are the most effective way to strengthen the pelvic floor muscles. These exercises involve repeatedly contracting and relaxing the muscles that stop the flow of urine. Kegel exercises can be done anywhere and at any time, such as when you're sitting at your desk or watching TV.

What is the pelvic diaphragm also known as?

The pelvic floor, or pelvic diaphragm, is a complex network of muscles, ligaments, and connective tissue that extends from the pubic bone to the tailbone. This system of muscles and tissue supports the pelvic organs (bladder, uterus, and rectum) and helps to keep them in place. The pelvic floor also plays an important role in sexual function and urinary continence. The pelvic floor muscles are often referred to as the "levator ani". These muscles span the opening of the pelvis and help to support the pelvic organs. The levator ani muscles are divided into three groups: the pubococcygeus, the iliococcygeus, and the coccygeus. The pubococcygeus muscle is the largest and most important of the pelvic floor muscles. This muscle forms a "hammock" that supports the pelvic organs. It also helps to close the urethra, the vagina, and the anus. The iliococcygeus muscle is a small, triangular muscle that attaches to the side of the pelvis. This muscle helps to support the pelvic organs and to keep them in place. The coccygeus muscle is a small, triangular muscle that attaches to the tailbone. This muscle helps to support the pelvic organs and to keep them in place. The pelvic floor muscles work together to support the pelvic organs and to keep them in place. These muscles also help to control urination and defecation.

What are the symptoms of a damaged diaphragm?

Symptoms of a damaged diaphragm may include: - Shortness of breath - Chest pain - Difficulty speaking - Difficulty swallowing - Pain with movement - Muscle weakness A damaged diaphragm can cause a number of symptoms that may make it difficult to breathe or speak. The diaphragm is a large, flat muscle that lies between the chest and abdomen. It is the primary muscle used for breathing. When the diaphragm is damaged, it may not be able to function properly. This can lead to shortness of breath, chest pain, difficulty speaking, difficulty swallowing, pain with movement, and muscle weakness.

In conclusion, the pelvic floor is a very important muscle group that can often be overlooked. It is responsible for many functions, including urinary and fecal continence, sexual function, and support of the abdominal and pelvic organs. When the pelvic floor muscles are weak, there can be many negative consequences, such as incontinence, sexual dysfunction, and hernias. It is important to keep the pelvic floor muscles strong by doing exercises such as Kegels.

What weakens pelvic floor muscles?

The pelvic floor muscles can be weakened by a variety of things. One common reason is pregnancy and childbirth. The extra weight of the baby and the increased pressure on the pelvic floor can weaken the muscles.

Other reasons can include chronic cough, constipation, and obesity. When the pelvic floor muscles are weakened, it can lead to a condition called pelvic organ prolapse. This is when the organs in the pelvis (including the uterus, vagina, bladder, and rectum) drop down from their normal position and bulge into or out of the vagina. This can cause symptoms such as urinary leakage, pelvic pain, and difficulty emptying the bladder or bowels. Pelvic organ prolapse is more common in women who have had multiple pregnancies, are older, or have other risk factors such as being overweight or having a family history of the condition. Fortunately, there are treatments available to help women with pelvic organ prolapse. These can include pelvic floor muscle exercises, weight loss, and surgery.

What is the best sleeping position for tight pelvic floor?

There is no definitive answer to this question as different people have different preferences. Some people find that sleeping on their back with a pillow under their knees can help to relieve pressure on the pelvic floor, while others find that sleeping on their side with a pillow between their legs is more comfortable. There are also many other possible sleeping positions that may be helpful for people with a tight pelvic floor. Some people may need to experiment with different positions to find the one that works best for them.

What does a tight pelvic floor feel like?

When your pelvic floor muscles are strong and tight, you may not be able to feel them. But when these muscles are weak, you may notice a difference in how you feel. For example, you may have: -Leakage of urine or stool when you cough, laugh, or sneeze -An inability to control the timing or amount of urine or stool -A feeling of heaviness in your pelvic area -A feeling of fullness in your rectum -Aching in your pelvic area or rectum

-Pain during sex If you have any of these symptoms, it doesn't necessarily mean that you have a weak pelvic floor. Other conditions can cause these symptoms. But it's worth talking to your doctor about how you're feeling. Weakness in your pelvic floor muscles can be caused by: -Pregnancy -Childbirth -A sedentary lifestyle -Being overweight -Chronic coughing -Constipation -A pelvic injury Fortunately, there are things you can do to strengthen your pelvic floor muscles. Kegel exercises are one option. These exercises involve repeatedly contracting and relaxing the muscles that you use to control urine flow. You can do Kegel exercises anywhere and at any time. Another option is pelvic floor physical therapy. This type of therapy can help you learn how to properly contract and relax your pelvic floor muscles. It can also help you identify and correct any other factors that may be contributing to your symptoms. If you're dealing with weak pelvic floor muscles, there's no need to feel embarrassed or ashamed. These problems are relatively common and can be very frustrating. But there are treatment options available. Talk to your doctor about what might be best for you.

Does walking relax the pelvic floor?

It is a common misconception that walking – or any type of exercise, for that matter – can relax the pelvic floor. The pelvic floor is a group of muscles, ligaments, and connective tissue that forms a bowl-like structure at the base of the pelvis. These muscles support the pelvic organs and help to control urinary and bowel function. The pelvic floor muscles can be thought of as a hammock, with the bottom of the pelvis being the “seat” of the hammock. The pelvic floor muscles can become tight or weak due to a variety of factors, such as pregnancy, childbirth, age, obesity, and inactivity. When these muscles are weak, it can lead to problems such as incontinence (leakage of urine or feces), pelvic organ prolapse (when the pelvic organs droop or bulge into the vagina), and sexual dysfunction. There are a number of pelvic floor exercises that can help to strengthen these muscles, but walking is not one of them. Walking is a great exercise for overall fitness and health, but it does not specifically target the pelvic floor muscles. If you are concerned about the health of your pelvic floor, it is best to consult with a doctor or pelvic floor physical therapist. They can help to assess your individual needs and recommend the best course of action, whether that includes exercises, lifestyle changes, or other treatments.

Is it ever too late to start pelvic floor exercises?

It is never too late to start pelvic floor exercises! Whether you are postpartum, perimenopausal, or post-menopausal, these exercises can help improve your pelvic floor health. Pelvic floor exercises, also known as Kegels, are not just for pregnant women or new mothers. Kegels can help improve bladder control, sexual function, and help prevent prolapse. If you are postpartum, pelvic floor exercises can help your body heal and recover from childbirth. Childbirth can weaken the pelvic floor muscles, so it is important to start doing Kegels as soon as possible post-delivery. If you are perimenopausal or post-menopausal, you may be experiencing changes in your body such as vaginal dryness, hot flashes, or night sweats. Kegel exercises can help improve sexual function, vaginal health, and overall pelvic floor health during these changes. To do a Kegel, simply squeeze the muscles you would use to stop the flow of urine. Hold for a count of 10, and then relax for a count of 10. Repeat this 10 times, 3 times a day. Kegel exercises are easy to do and can be done anywhere, at any time. So there's no excuse not to start today!

What is the best position to do pelvic floor exercises?

There are a few different schools of thought when it comes to the best position to do pelvic floor exercises. Some say that it is best to do them lying down, so that you can fully relax your muscles and focus on the exercise. Others say that it is best to do them sitting up, so that you can maintain good posture and engage your core muscles. And still others say that it is best to do them standing up, so that you can use gravity to your advantage. So, which is the best position to do pelvic floor exercises? The answer may depend on your individual situation and what your goals are. If you are just starting out, it may be best to do them lying down, so that you can get a feeling for the muscles involved and focus on the exercise. If you are trying to improve your posture, it may be best to do them sitting up. And if you are trying to increase your strength, it may be best to do them standing up. Ultimately, the best position to do pelvic floor exercises is the one that works best for you. If you are not sure where to start, you can always consult with a physical therapist or other healthcare professional to get personalized advice.

What are the 4 diaphragms of the body?

There are four diaphragms in the human body: the pelvic floor, the respiratory diaphragm, the cardiovascular diaphragm, and the reproductive diaphragm. The pelvic floor is a muscular and fibrous structure that spans the bottom of the pelvis. It supports the pelvic organs and helps to keep them in place. The pelvic floor is also responsible for bowel and bladder control. The respiratory diaphragm is a dome-shaped muscle that separates the chest cavity from the abdominal cavity. It contracts and relaxes during breathing to help move air in and out of the lungs. The cardiovascular diaphragm is a muscular structure that separates the heart from the lungs. It helps to pump blood from the heart and into the lungs. The reproductive diaphragm is a muscular and fibrous structure that spans the pelvis. It helps to support the reproductive organs and keep them in place.

The pelvic floor is an essential part of the female reproductive system, and it is important to keep it healthy and functioning properly. There are a number of ways to do this, including regular exercise, avoiding tobacco and excess alcohol, and maintaining a healthy weight. If you think you may have a problem with your pelvic floor, talk to your doctor.

Can you repair a damaged diaphragm?

The diaphragm is a thin, flat muscle that lies at the bottom of the ribcage. It is the muscle that helps you breathe in and out. When you breathe in, the diaphragm contracts and pulls air into your lungs. When you breathe out, the diaphragm relaxes and pushes the air out of your lungs. The diaphragm can be damaged by surgery, radiation therapy, or other injuries. This can cause problems with breathing. If the diaphragm is damaged, it can be repaired. Surgery is the most common treatment. The doctor will make an incision in your chest and put the diaphragm back in place. The surgery can be done through a large incision (open surgery) or a small incision (laparoscopic surgery). After surgery, you will likely need to stay in the hospital for a few days. You will also need to take it easy for several weeks. You will likely need physical therapy to help you regain your strength. The success of surgery depends on the severity of the damage. In most cases, the diaphragm can be repaired. But, in some cases, the damage may be too severe and surgery may not be an option. If you have damage to your diaphragm, talk to your doctor about your treatment options.

What does diaphragm pain feel like?

The pelvic floor is a group of muscles that support the pelvic organs, including the bladder, uterus, and rectum. These muscles are located between the legs, running from the pubic bone to the tailbone. The pelvic floor muscles help to control urination and bowel movements, and they also help to support the pelvic organs during pregnancy and childbirth. Diaphragm pain can feel like a sharp, dull, or burning pain in the pelvic area. The pain may be constant or it may come and go. The pain may be worse with certain activities, such as sitting for long periods of time, coughing, or sneezing. Diaphragm pain may also be worse during menstruation. The cause of diaphragm pain is often unknown. However, the pain may be related to an injury or condition that affects the pelvic floor muscles, such as pelvic floor muscle spasm, pelvic floor muscle tension, or pelvic inflammatory disease. Treatment for diaphragm pain typically includes home remedies, such as heat therapy and over-the-counter pain medication. In some cases, additional treatment may be necessary, such as physical therapy or surgery.

What causes diaphragm problems?

There are a variety of possible causes for diaphragm problems. Some of the more common causes include: Muscle fatigue: The diaphragm is a muscle, and like any muscle, it can become tired and sore with overuse. This is often seen in athletes or other people who engage in strenuous activities on a regular basis. Dehydration: Dehydration can cause the diaphragm to cramp and spasm, making it difficult to contract and relax properly. Injury: An injury to the diaphragm, whether from a car accident or another type of trauma, can cause it to malfunction. Nerve damage: Damage to the nerves that control the diaphragm can also lead to diaphragm problems. This can be caused by diseases like ALS or Parkinson's, or by injuries to the spinal cord or other parts of the nervous system. Surgery: Surgery on the lungs or other organs in the chest can sometimes damage the diaphragm, leading to problems. Pregnancy: The growing uterus can put pressure on the diaphragm and interfere with its normal functioning. This is usually only a temporary problem, but in some cases the diaphragm may not return to its pre-pregnancy state. Obesity: Extra weight can put pressure on the diaphragm and make it harder for it to contract and relax properly.

Smoking: Smoking can irritate and inflame the diaphragm, and has also been linked to an increased risk of diaphragm cancer.

Does diaphragm weaken with age?

As we age, our bodies go through a lot of changes. We may not be as strong as we once were, and our balance may not be what it used to be. One thing that can change as we age is the condition of our pelvic floor. The pelvic floor is a group of muscles and tissues that support the bladder and other organs in the pelvis. These muscles can weaken over time, which can lead to incontinence and other problems. There are a number of things that can cause the pelvic floor to weaken, including pregnancy, childbirth, and menopause. Age can also be a factor. There are a few things you can do to help keep your pelvic floor strong. Kegel exercises are one option. These exercises help to strengthen the pelvic floor muscles. You can also try to avoid things that can weaken the pelvic floor, such as lifting heavy objects, coughing or sneezing without using proper technique, and jumping or running without warmup. If you think you may have a problem with your pelvic floor, talk to your doctor. There are treatments available that can help.

What kind of doctor treats the diaphragm?

Your diaphragm is a large, dome-shaped muscle that separates your chest from your abdomen. It's an important muscle for breathing, and it also plays a role in keeping your guts in place. When something goes wrong with your diaphragm, it can be very uncomfortable. There are a few different types of doctors who can treat problems with your diaphragm. If you have a serious injury to your diaphragm, you will likely be seen by a surgeon. Surgeons can repair tears or holes in your diaphragm. In some cases, they may need to remove part of your diaphragm. If you have an infection in your diaphragm, you will be treated by an infectious disease specialist. This type of doctor is an expert in treating infections. If you have a problem with the nerves that control your diaphragm, you may be seen by a neurologist. Neurologists are doctors who specialize in treating problems with the nervous system. If you have a problem with the way your diaphragm is shaped, you may be seen by a cardiothoracic surgeon. These surgeons specialize in operating on the heart, lungs, and chest. You may also be seen by a gastroenterologist if you have a problem with your diaphragm. Gastroenterologists are doctors who specialize in treating problems with the digestive system.

What happens if your diaphragm is weak?

A weak diaphragm can have many consequences, some of which may be quite serious. When the diaphragm is weak, it cannot effectively push down on the abdominal contents, which can lead to a number of problems. One of the most common problems associated with a weak diaphragm is hiatal hernia. This occurs when the stomach protrudes through the diaphragm and into the chest cavity. This can cause a number of symptoms, including heartburn, chest pain, and difficulty swallowing. Another common problem is gastroparesis, which is a condition where the stomach muscles are not able to effectively contract and move food along. This can lead to nausea, vomiting, and bloating. In some cases, a weak diaphragm can also lead to difficulty breathing. This is because the diaphragm is responsible for helping to move air in and out of the lungs. If it is not working properly, it can result in shortness of breath and difficulty getting enough oxygen into the blood. If you have a weak diaphragm, it is important to see a doctor so that they can determine the cause and develop a treatment plan. In some cases, a simple exercise program can help to strengthen the diaphragm and improve its function. In other cases, more aggressive treatment may be necessary, such as surgery.

Can poor posture affect your diaphragm?

When you think of good posture, you might think of standing up straight with your shoulders back. But did you know that good posture starts from the ground up? Your feet should be shoulder-width apart, your knees should be slightly bent, and your pelvis should be in a neutral position. This may feel like you're sticking your butt out, but it's actually the best way to align your spine. Your diaphragm is a large muscle that sits at the base of your lungs and is essential for breathing. When you breathe in, your diaphragm contracts and moves downward, pushing your abdominal contents down and out of the way. This increases the amount of space in your chest cavity, and allows your lungs to expand and fill with air. When you have good posture, your diaphragm is able to move more efficiently. However, when you have poor posture, your diaphragm can become constricted. This can make it more difficult to breathe, and can also lead to pain in your back, neck, and shoulders. So, how can you improve your posture? Start by standing up straight and tall. Make sure your feet are shoulder-width apart and your knees are slightly bent. Tuck your chin slightly and relax your shoulders. Once you've found your neutral pelvis position, try to maintain it throughout the day. This may take some practice, but it's worth it! Good posture not only helps your diaphragm to work more efficiently, but it can also help to prevent pain in your back, neck, and shoulders. So, next time you're standing or sitting, make sure to check your posture. It may just be the key to deep, pain-free breaths.

The pelvic floor is a group of muscles and ligaments that support the pelvic organs and span the bony pelvis. The pelvic floor muscles are the levator ani and coccygeus muscles. The pelvic floor muscles attach to the pelvis at the pubic bone, ischial spine, and sacrum. The pelvic floor muscles support the pelvic organs, including the bladder, uterus, and rectum. The levator ani muscle is the primary muscle of the pelvic floor and is responsible for supporting the pelvic organs and maintaining continence. The coccygeus muscle is responsible for stabilizing the sacrum and the ischial spine. Pelvic floor muscle training (PFMT) is an effective treatment for urinary incontinence and can be used to prevent or treat pelvic floor disorders.

What causes weak pelvic floor?

Pelvic floor weakness can have many different causes. Childbirth, surgery, and ageing are all potential causes of weakened pelvic floor muscles. Childbirth is often the cause of weak pelvic floor muscles. The process of childbirth can cause the pelvic floor muscles to become stretched and damaged. This can lead to a loss of muscle tone and a decrease in the ability to control the muscles of the pelvis. Surgery can also damage the pelvic floor muscles. Operations involving the pelvis, such as a hysterectomy, can damage the muscles and nerves of the pelvic floor. ageing can also cause the pelvic floor muscles to weaken. As we age, the muscles of the body begin to lose some of their strength and tone. This can lead to a loss of control over the pelvic floor muscles and may cause them to become weak. There are many different treatments for weak pelvic floor muscles. Physical therapy is often used to help strengthen and tone the muscles. In some cases, surgery may be needed to repair damage to the muscles or to correct a structural problem. Pelvic floor exercises, such as Kegels, can also help to strengthen the muscles and improve muscle control.

How long does it take to strengthen your pelvic floor?

It takes anywhere from 2-6 weeks to see any strengthening of your pelvic floor muscles. Even then, only about 30% of women report feeling stronger after 6 weeks. Your best bet is to keep at it, and continue with pelvic floor muscle exercises of some kind for at least 3-6 months. After that time, you can start to ease off a bit, but it is still a good idea to do some form of pelvic floor muscle exercise on a regular basis (weekly or monthly, for example) for the rest of your life.

What does a weak pelvic floor feel like?

A weak pelvic floor can feel like a lot of things. For some, it might feel like they're constantly leaking urine or stool. Others might feel like they can't control their bowels or bladder. Some might even feel like they're going to lose control of their bowel or bladder at any given moment. For some people, a weak pelvic floor can also cause pain during sex. This is because the pelvic floor muscles help to support the uterus, bladder, and rectum. If these muscles are weak, it can lead to pain during sex. There are also a number of other symptoms that can be associated with a weak pelvic floor. These include: - Urinary incontinence - fecal incontinence - Painful sex - Pelvic organ prolapse - Lower back pain - Joint pain If you're experiencing any of these symptoms, it's important to see a doctor. They can help to determine if your pelvic floor is weak and recommend treatment options.

How do you know if your pelvic floor is weak?

The pelvic floor is a group of muscles and ligaments that form a bowl-shaped sling at the bottom of the pelvis. These muscles and ligaments support the bladder and intestines, and during pregnancy and childbirth, they also support the weight of the growing baby. Over time, the pelvic floor muscles can weaken due to pregnancy, childbirth, age, weight gain, and other factors. This can lead to a condition called pelvic floor dysfunction (PFD), which can cause urinary incontinence, fecal incontinence, and pelvic organ prolapse. There are several symptoms that may indicate that your pelvic floor is weak or damaged. If you experience any of the following, you should see your doctor for an evaluation: - urinary incontinence (leaking urine when you cough, sneeze, or laugh) - difficulty urinating or holding back urine - fecal incontinence (leaking stool) - pelvic organ prolapse (feeling like your uterus, bladder, or rectum is falling out of your vagina) - pain during sex - pain in the pelvic area - muscle spasms in the pelvic floor muscles

Can you reverse a weak pelvic floor?

The pelvic floor is a group of muscles located at the bottom of the pelvis that support the bladder, uterus, and rectum. The pelvic floor muscles are important for urinary continence, sexual function, and childbirth. A weak pelvic floor can cause urinary incontinence, sexual dysfunction, and prolapse of organs. There are many factors that can contribute to a weak pelvic floor, including pregnancy, childbirth, menopause, and chronic conditions such as obesity and constipation. Pelvic floor exercises, also known as Kegels, are the most effective way to strengthen the pelvic floor muscles. Kegels can be done anywhere, at any time, and do not require any special equipment. To do a Kegel, simply squeeze the pelvic floor muscles as if you are trying to stop urinating midstream. Hold the contraction for 5-10 seconds and then relax for 5 seconds. Repeat 10-20 times. For some people, Kegels alone are enough to reverse a weak pelvic floor. Others may need to combine Kegels with other treatments, such as weight loss or medications. Surgery is rarely needed to treat a weak pelvic floor. If you are experiencing urinary incontinence, sexual dysfunction, or prolapse of organs, talk to your doctor about whether pelvic floor exercises are right for you.

How common is weak pelvic floor?

It's estimated that as many as one in three women experience weak pelvic floor muscles. The pelvic floor is a group of muscles that support the bladder, uterus, and rectum. They can become weak due to pregnancy, childbirth, and aging. Weak pelvic floor muscles can lead to urinary incontinence, fecal incontinence, and prolapse of the uterus or rectum. There are several factors that can contribute to weak pelvic floor muscles. Pregnancy and childbirth are two of the most common causes. The added weight of the baby and the strain of childbirth can weaken the pelvic floor muscles. Aging can also lead to weakened pelvic floor muscles. The loss of estrogen after menopause can cause the pelvic floor muscles to become thinner and less strong. There are several treatments available for weak pelvic floor muscles. Kegel exercises are often recommended to help strengthen the muscles. Pelvic floor physical therapy can also be helpful. In some cases, surgery may be necessary to correct the problem. If you are experiencing any urinary or fecal incontinence, or prolapse of the uterus or rectum, it is important to see your doctor. Weak pelvic floor muscles can be treated, and there is no need to suffer in silence.

What does a strong pelvic floor feel like?

When we think about the pelvic floor, we often think about kegel exercises and preventing incontinence. However, having a strong pelvic floor can offer so much more than that! A strong pelvic floor can lead to improved sexual function, increased sensation during sex, and more. So, what does a strong pelvic floor feel like? For women, a strong pelvic floor feels like increased sensation and tightness during sex. It can also lead to more intense orgasms. For men, a strong pelvic floor can lead to improved erections and more control over ejaculation. In both sexes, a strong pelvic floor can lead to an improved overall sex life. So how do you know if you have a strong pelvic floor? One way to find out is to consult with a pelvic floor physical therapist. They can help to assess your pelvic floor strength and offer advice on how to improve it. There are also at-home tests you can do to get an idea of your pelvic floor strength. One simple test is the "stop and start" test. To do this, start urinating and then try to stop mid-stream. If you can stop urinating without losing control, then you have a good pelvic floor. Another test is the "kegel" test. This involves tightening the muscles around the anus and vagina as if you were trying to stop urinating. If you can hold the muscles tight for 10 seconds, then you have a good pelvic floor. If you're not sure about your pelvic floor strength, or if you want to improve it, there are a few things you can do. Kegel exercises are one way to improve the strength of your pelvic floor. These involve repeatedly contracting and relaxing the muscles around the anus and vagina. You can also try using pelvic floor muscle trainers, which are devices that help to strengthen the muscles. Having a strong pelvic floor can offer many benefits, both sexually and non-sexually. If you're interested in learning more about the pelvic floor and how to strengthen it, speak to a pelvic floor physical therapist or consult with your doctor.

The pelvic floor is a group of muscles, ligaments, and connective tissues that support the bladder, uterus, and rectum. The pelvic floor also helps to close off the urethra and vagina. The pelvic floor is important for both men and women, but it is especially important for women during pregnancy and childbirth. Pelvic floor problems can cause incontinence, pelvic pain, and sexual dysfunction. There are many treatments available for pelvic floor problems, and most can be effectively treated with physical therapy.

How do you test if you have a strong pelvic floor?

There are a few ways that you can test if you have a strong pelvic floor. One way is to see if you can stop your urine stream while you are urinating. If you are able to do this, it is likely that you have a strong pelvic floor. Another way to test is to place a finger in your vagina and see if you can feel a muscle contract when you try to squeeze it. If you can, then you probably have a strong pelvic floor. If you want to be sure, you can always consult with a doctor or pelvic floor physiotherapist. They will be able to give you a more thorough examination and let you know for sure whether or not you have a strong pelvic floor. Having a strong pelvic floor is important for many reasons. For one, it can help to prevent incontinence. This is when urine leaks out unexpectedly. A strong pelvic floor can also help to make sex more enjoyable by providing more support and sensation. Additionally, a strong pelvic floor can help to reduce the risk of prolapse. This is when organs in the pelvic area fall out of place. There are many things that you can do to help strengthen your pelvic floor. One is to do special exercises called Kegels. These are when you squeeze the muscles in your pelvic floor as if you were trying to stop the flow of urine. You can also try to incorporate some pelvic floor muscle training into your regular workout routine. For example, when you are doing squats, you can try to hold in your pelvic floor muscles as you lower yourself down. If you are concerned about your pelvic floor, or if you are experiencing any problems with incontinence or prolapse, be sure to consult with a doctor or pelvic floor physiotherapist. They will be able to help you figure out the best way to strengthen your pelvic floor and improve your overall health.

Can a virgin have weak pelvic floor?

A virgin is someone who has not had sexual intercourse. While there are many virgins out there, there is no medical definition for the term. In order to have weak pelvic floor muscles, one would need to have some sort of pelvic floor dysfunction. There are many things that can cause pelvic floor dysfunction, including but not limited to:

- childbirth

- being overweight or obese

- chronic coughing or constipation

- age-related changes

While it is possible for a virgin to have weak pelvic floor muscles, it is not likely. The pelvic floor is a group of muscles that support the pelvis and keep it in place. These muscles are usually very strong and can only be weakened by things like childbirth or chronic coughing. So, while it is

Should I go to the doctor for weak pelvic floor?

If you are experiencing any kind of pelvic floor dysfunction, it is important to seek out medical help. This is because pelvic floor dysfunction can lead to a number of different health problems, including urinary incontinence, fecal incontinence, and even pelvic organ prolapse. There are a number of different treatments available for pelvic floor dysfunction, and the best course of treatment will vary depending on the individual. However, some simple lifestyle changes can often help to improve the condition, and pelvic floor physical therapy is often recommended as a first-line treatment option. If you are experiencing any symptoms of pelvic floor dysfunction, it is important to speak to your doctor so that they can assess your individual situation and offer the best treatment option for you.

What exercises strengthen your pelvic floor?

When we think of exercising to improve our pelvic floor, we often think of Kegel exercises. However, there are many other exercises that can help to improve the strength of your pelvic floor. These include: - Pilates: Pilates is a great way to strengthen your core, which in turn will help to support your pelvic floor. - Yoga: Yoga can help to improve your overall flexibility and muscle tone, both of which are important for the health of your pelvic floor. - Squats: Squats are a great way to work the muscles of your lower body, including those in your pelvic floor. - Lunges: Like squats, lunges work the muscles of your lower body, including your pelvic floor. - Bridging: Bridging is an excellent way to target the muscles of your glutes and lower back, both of which can help to support your pelvic floor. These are just a few examples of the many exercises that can help to improve the strength of your pelvic floor. Talk to your doctor or a physical therapist to find out which exercises would be best for you.

What does a pelvic floor physiotherapist do?

A pelvic floor physiotherapist is a specialist who helps people with problems in the muscles and connective tissues of the pelvis. The pelvic floor is the group of muscles and tissues that support the bladder, rectum, and uterus. Problems with the pelvic floor can lead to urinary or fecal incontinence, pelvic pain, and sexual dysfunction. Pelvic floor physiotherapy can help to improve or resolve these problems. The physiotherapist will assess the pelvic floor muscles and tissues, and develop a treatment plan based on the findings. This may include exercises to improve muscle strength and flexibility, techniques to improve coordination and control of the muscles, and education on how to reduce or avoid activities that may aggravate the problem.

There are many things that can be done to improve pelvic floor health. kegel exercises are one method that can be used to strengthen the pelvic floor muscles. Other things that can be done to improve pelvic floor health include avoiding constipation and managing stress.

How long does it take to restore your pelvic floor?

It is difficult to say how long it will take to fully restore your pelvic floor. This is because it depends on the level of damage, how well you follow your rehabilitation plan, and your overall health. That being said, it is important to give yourself enough time to heal and fully restore your pelvic floor. This is a sensitive area of your body and rushing the healing process can lead to further damage or even longer healing times. If you have experienced pelvic floor damage, it is important to consult with a pelvic floor physiotherapist. They will be able to assess the level of damage and develop a rehabilitation plan that is tailored to your needs. They will also be able to give you a more accurate estimate of how long it will take to heal. In general, it takes several weeks to a few months to see significant improvements in the pelvic floor. However, it can take up to a year or more to fully restore the pelvic floor. This is why it is so important to be patient and follow your rehabilitation plan. If you are experiencing pelvic floor problems, don't hesitate to seek help. There are many resources available and you don't have to go through this alone.

Does lifting weights tighten pelvic floor?

Lifting weights is often touted as a way to tighten and tone the body, but can it really help with pelvic floor problems? The pelvic floor is a group of muscles, ligaments and tissues that provides support for the pelvic organs. These muscles can become weak or damaged due to pregnancy, childbirth, age, obesity and other factors. This can lead to incontinence, prolapse and other pelvic floor disorders. There is some evidence that lifting weights can help to strengthen the pelvic floor muscles and improve incontinence. A 2012 study found that pelvic floor muscle training (PFMT) was effective in improving incontinence in overweight and obese women. A 2013 study also found that PFMT was effective in treating stress incontinence in post-menopausal women. Lifting weights is not the only way to strengthen the pelvic floor muscles. Other exercises, such as Kegels, can also be effective. However, lifting weights may be a good option for those who are unable to do other exercises, or who want to add some variety to their routine. If you are considering adding weightlifting to your exercise routine, be sure to talk to your doctor first. They can help you develop a safe and effective workout plan.

Does weak pelvic floor cause weak glutes?

The pelvic floor is a group of muscles and tissues that form a sling at the bottom of the pelvis. These muscles and tissues support the bladder and the bowels, and they help to control the release of urine and feces. The pelvic floor muscles also help to support the uterus and the vagina. Some experts believe that weak pelvic floor muscles can lead to weak glutes. The reason for this is that the pelvic floor muscles and the gluteal muscles are both connected to the pelvis. When the pelvic floor muscles are weak, they can't provide the same level of support for the pelvis. This can lead to instability in the pelvis, and this can eventually lead to weak glutes. There is some evidence that weak pelvic floor muscles can lead to weak glutes. For example, one study found that women with weak pelvic floor muscles were more likely to have weak gluteal muscles. However, this does not necessarily mean that weak pelvic floor muscles cause weak glutes. It is possible that both conditions are caused by another underlying factor. Weak glutes can cause a number of problems, including lower back pain, knee pain, and hip pain. Weak pelvic floor muscles can also lead to urinary incontinence and prolapse of the bladder or the uterus. If you are experiencing any of these problems, it is important to see a doctor to rule out other potential causes. If you have weak pelvic floor muscles, there are a number of things you can do to strengthen them. pelvic floor muscle exercises, also known as Kegel exercises, are one option. You can also try using a pelvic floor muscle toner or biofeedback device. These devices can help to increase the strength of your pelvic floor muscles.

How do you tell if your bladder has fallen?

There are a few key signs that may indicate that a person has a prolapsed bladder. The first is if they feel a sensation of heaviness or fullness in their pelvis, as well as a feeling of pressure in the vagina. They may also notice that their urine stream has become weaker, and that they are urinating more frequently than usual. In some cases, a prolapsed bladder can also cause constipation. If you think you may have a prolapsed bladder, it is important to see a doctor so that they can rule out other possible causes of your symptoms. They will likely carry out a physical examination, which may involve inserting a gloved finger into your vagina to check for prolapse. They may also order an ultrasound scan or a cystoscopy, which is a procedure where a thin, flexible tube is inserted into the bladder through the urethra so that the doctor can get a better view of the bladder.

The pelvic floor is a group of muscles, ligaments, and connective tissue that stretch across the bottom of the pelvis. These muscles and tissues support the organs in the pelvis, including the bladder, uterus, and rectum. The pelvic floor also helps to control the release of urine and feces. The pelvic floor is an important part of the body that helps to support the organs in the pelvis and control the release of urine and feces. These muscles and tissues can be weakened by pregnancy, childbirth, and aging, which can lead to problems such as urinary incontinence. Pelvic floor exercises can help to strengthen the muscles and improve the function of the pelvic floor.

Can a pelvic exam tell if you are a virgin?

A pelvic exam is usually done as part of a woman's regular checkup. It is a way for doctors to check on the health of a woman's reproductive organs. The exam can also tell if a woman is pregnant. A pelvic exam is not a test to see if someone is a virgin. virginity is not medical condition.

During a pelvic exam, the doctor inserts two gloved fingers into the vagina. They also press on the lower abdomen with the other hand. This allows them to feel theShape, size, and position of the uterus and ovaries. The doctor may also take a sample of tissue from the vagina or cervix to test for infection.

A pelvic exam can be a little uncomfortable, but it should not be painful. If it is, tell the doctor.Some women feel more comfortable if they put their legs in stirrups. This spreads the vaginal walls and gives the doctor a clear view.

Pelvic exams are an important part of preventative health care for women. They help catch problems early, when they are more easily treated.

What are the most common pelvic floor disorders?

The most common pelvic floor disorders are: 1. Pelvic organ prolapse: This occurs when the pelvic organs (bladder, uterus, rectum, or small intestine) drop down from their normal position and protrude into or outside of the vagina. 2. Urinary incontinence: This is leakage of urine from the bladder. It can be caused by weak muscles or nerves around the bladder. 3. Fecal incontinence: This is leakage of stool from the rectum. It can be caused by weak muscles or nerves around the rectum. 4. Painful intercourse: This can be caused by vaginal atrophy (thinning and drying of the vaginal walls), vaginal stenosis (narrowing of the vagina), or other pelvic floor disorders. 5. Urinary urgency and frequency: This can be caused by an overactive bladder, which can be a symptom of another pelvic floor disorder. 6. Difficulty emptying the bladder or bowel: This can be caused by blockages in the urinary or digestive tracts, or by weak muscles in the pelvic floor.

How can I strengthen my pelvic floor naturally?

The pelvic floor is a hammock of muscles, ligaments and tissues that span the bottom of the pelvis. The pelvic floor supports the bladder and bowel in men, and the uterus and vagina in women. The pelvic floor muscles contract and relax to control the flow of urine and feces. Pelvic floor muscles can weaken with age, pregnancy and childbirth, and from carrying extra weight. Weak pelvic floor muscles can lead to incontinence, a condition in which you can't control your urine or feces. You can do pelvic floor muscle exercises (Kegels) to strengthen your pelvic floor muscles. Kegels are easy to do, and you can do them anywhere, anytime. To do a Kegel, squeeze the muscles you would use to stop the flow of urine. Hold the squeeze for three to five seconds, then relax for five seconds. Repeat 10 to 15 times. As your muscles get stronger, you can hold the squeeze longer. You may feel your muscles working, but if you don't, try this: Sit on the toilet with your knees apart. Place your hand on your stomach just below your navel. Slowly tighten your stomach muscles, bringing your navel toward your spine. At the same time, tighten the muscles in your lower pelvis as if you are trying to stop the flow of urine. Now, let go of your stomach muscles and relax the muscles in your pelvis. You should feel your pelvic floor muscles relax and your stomach muscles loosen. If you're having trouble locating your pelvic floor muscles, think about them as the muscles you use to stop the flow of urine. Once you've found them, you can do Kegels anywhere, anytime — in the car, at work, even while you're watching TV. Kegels are not just for women. Men can also benefit from doing Kegels to strengthen their pelvic floor muscles. Kegels can help men who have incontinence or who want to prevent incontinence. Kegels can also help men with erectile dysfunction by increasing blood flow to the penis. If you're doing Kegels and still leaking urine, talk to your doctor.You may have a more serious problem, such as a prolapsed bladder.

Can you fix pelvic floor dysfunction at home?

Pelvic floor dysfunction is a common condition that can affect both men and women. The pelvic floor is a group of muscles that support the pelvis and help to control bowel and bladder function. When these muscles are weak or too tight, they can cause problems with urination, defecation, and sexual function. There are a number of ways to treat pelvic floor dysfunction, but can it be fixed at home? The answer is yes and no. Some simple lifestyle changes can help to improve the condition, but more serious cases may require professional help. One of the best things you can do for your pelvic floor is to maintain a healthy weight. Excess weight can put additional pressure on the muscles and lead to further weakening. If you are overweight, losing even a few pounds can have a significant impact on your pelvic floor. Another important step is to avoid constipation. Constipation can put extra strain on the pelvic floor muscles and lead to further weakening. To avoid constipation, make sure to eat a high-fiber diet and drink plenty of fluids. If you are still having trouble, there are a number of over-the-counter laxatives that can help. There are also a number of exercises that can help to strengthen the pelvic floor muscles. These exercises can be done at home and do not require any special equipment. One simple exercise is to sit on the floor with your knees bent and your feet flat on the ground. Squeeze your pelvic floor muscles and hold for five seconds. Release and repeat 10 times. If you are still experiencing symptoms of pelvic floor dysfunction after making lifestyle changes and doing pelvic floor exercises, you may need to see a doctor. A number of treatments are available, including physical therapy, medication, and surgery.

When should you see a pelvic floor physiotherapist?

A pelvic floor physiotherapist can help to treat a wide range of pelvic floor disorders. The most common reason to see a pelvic floor physiotherapist is for incontinence (leakage of urine or faeces), prolapse (descent of organs from their normal position), or pain in the pelvic region. Other reasons may include postnatal incontinence or prolapse, post-operative incontinence or prolapse, and sexual dysfunction. It is important to note that not all pelvic floor problems will require specialist treatment, and often simple lifestyle and behaviour changes can make a big difference. However, if you are experiencing any of the above symptoms, it is recommended that you see a pelvic floor physiotherapist for assessment and treatment. During your initial consultation, your physiotherapist will take a detailed history and perform a physical examination. They will then be able to provide you with a diagnosis and treatment plan. Treatment may involve a combination of pelvic floor muscle exercises, manual therapy, electrical stimulation and education. If you are concerned about your pelvic floor health, the best thing to do is to see a pelvic floor physiotherapist for an assessment. They will be able to provide you with a diagnosis and treatment plan that is specific to your needs.

What is done during pelvic floor therapy?

During pelvic floor therapy, the therapist will work with the patient to assess and identify any areas of tightness, weakness, or imbalance. Once these areas have been identified, the therapist will work with the patient to release any tightness, strengthen any weaknesses, and restore balance to the pelvic floor muscles. Pelvic floor therapy can be done through a variety of methods, including manual release of tight muscles, exercises to strengthen weak muscles, and electrical stimulation to help balance the muscles.

Can squats damage your pelvic floor?

The pelvic floor is a group of muscles and ligaments that forms a bowl-shaped structure at the bottom of the pelvis. These muscles and ligaments provide support for the pelvic organs, including the bladder, rectum, and uterus. The pelvic floor also helps to control the release of urine and feces. There is some debate as to whether or not squats can damage the pelvic floor. One concern is that squats can put pressure on the bladder and cause urinary incontinence. Another worry is that deep squats can stretch or tear the pelvic floor muscles, leading to a condition called pelvic organ prolapse. So far, there is no definitive evidence that squats cause any damage to the pelvic floor. In fact, many experts believe that squats can actually help to strengthen the pelvic floor muscles. One study found that women who performed squats regularly had a lower risk of pelvic organ prolapse. If you are concerned about damaging your pelvic floor, you can speak to your doctor or a certified personal trainer. They can help you to choose the right exercises for your body and offer advice on how to avoid any potential injuries.

How does doctor check for pelvic floor dysfunction?

Doctors can check for pelvic floor dysfunction in a number of ways. One common method is called the "Q-tip test". This involves the doctor insert a Q-tip into the patient's vagina. They then measure the angle of the Q-tip. If the angle is greater than 30 degrees, it is considered a positive sign for pelvic floor dysfunction. Another common method is called the "finger test". This involves the doctor inserting a finger into the patient's vagina. They then feel for any bulges or weakness in the pelvic floor muscles. Both of these tests are relatively simple and can be done in a doctor's office. They can help to diagnose pelvic floor dysfunction and formulate a treatment plan.

Pelvic floor disorders are a common problem, especially for women. However, there are treatments available that can help. If you think you may have a pelvic floor disorder, talk to your doctor.

How do you massage your pelvic floor internally?

One way to massage your pelvic floor internally is to insert your fingers into your vagina and feel around for any knots or tension. You can also use a vibrator or other sex toy to massage your pelvic floor internally. Another way to massage your pelvic floor internally is to use your fingers to press on your G-spot or other sensitive areas. You may also want to try different positions to see what feels good. Experiment and find what works best for you!

Can a gynecologist treat pelvic floor dysfunction?

A pelvic floor disorder is a medical problem that affects a woman's ability to control her bowels, bladder, and uterus. The pelvic floor is a group of muscles, ligaments, and tissues that support these organs. While there are many different types of pelvic floor disorders, the most common one is pelvic floor dysfunction (PFD). PFD can cause a number of different symptoms, including: -Urinary incontinence (leaking urine) -Fecal incontinence (leaking stool) -Pelvic pain -Sexual dysfunction -Prolapse (when organs drop down into the vagina due to weakened muscles) While PFD can be a very debilitating condition, there is good news: it is treatable. And one of the best ways to treat PFD is to see a gynecologist who specializes in pelvic floor disorders. A gynecologist who specializes in pelvic floor disorders will be able to provide you with a comprehensive evaluation. This evaluation will include a thorough medical history and a physical exam. The gynecologist may also order additional tests, such as: -A urinary stress test: This test is used to assess for stress incontinence, which is the most common type of incontinence. During the test, you will be asked to cough or bearing down while a nurse monitors your urine output. -A cystometrogram: This test is used to assess for bladder dysfunction. During the test, a small catheter is inserted into your bladder and filled with fluid. The amount of urine your bladder can hold and how well it empties will be measured. -An electromyogram: This test is used to assess for pelvic floor muscle dysfunction. During the test, small needles will be inserted into your pelvic floor muscles. Electrical activity will be measured while you contract and relax your muscles. After the evaluation, the gynecologist will work with you to develop a treatment plan. The treatment plan will be individualized based on the type and severity of your symptoms. Treatment options may include: -Lifestyle changes: Many times, PFD can be managed with lifestyle changes, such as losing weight, avoiding constipation, and avoiding foods and beverages that irritate the bladder. -Pelvic floor muscle exercises: Pelvic floor muscle exercises, also known as Kegel exercises, can help to strengthen the muscles of the pelvic floor. This can help to improve or even eliminate symptoms. -Bladder training: Bladder training is a form of behavior therapy that can help to retrain the bladder. The goal of bladder training is to increase the amount of time between urination. -Medications: There are a number of different medications that can be used to treat PFD. These medications can help to relieve symptoms, such as urinary incontinence and pelvic pain. -Inject

When is it too late for Kegels?

The pelvic floor is a group of muscles and ligaments that support the pelvic organs, including the bladder, uterus, and rectum. The pelvic floor muscles are located between the pubic bone and the tailbone, and they contract and relax to allow urine and stool to pass through the urethra and anus. Kegels are exercises that strengthen the pelvic floor muscles. These exercises can be performed anywhere, at any time, and don't require any special equipment. Kegels can be beneficial for both men and women. They can help with urinary incontinence, pelvic organ prolapse, and sexual dysfunction. Most people can benefit from doing Kegels. However, there are some people who should not do Kegels. These people include: -People with pelvic floor muscle spasm or pelvic pain syndrome. -People who have had recent surgery in the pelvic area. -People who have had a pelvic floor injury, such as a perineal tear. If you're not sure if Kegels are right for you, talk to your doctor or pelvic floor physical therapist.

How do you fix pelvic floor dysfunction?

Pelvic floor dysfunction is a common problem that can cause a number of symptoms, including pain in the lower abdomen, difficult or painful urination, and pain during sexual intercourse. The pelvic floor is a group of muscles and tissues that support the uterus, bladder, and rectum, and when these muscles and tissues are not functioning properly, pelvic floor dysfunction can occur. There are a number of different ways to treat pelvic floor dysfunction, depending on the cause and severity of the problem. For mild cases of pelvic floor dysfunction, simple lifestyle changes may be enough to relieve symptoms. This can include things like avoiding constipation, which can put additional pressure on the pelvic floor muscles, and practicing regular Kegel exercises, which can help to strengthen the muscles. For more moderate to severe cases of pelvic floor dysfunction, there are a number of different therapies that can be used. Physical therapy is often used to help reduce pain and increase muscle strength and flexibility. Biofeedback and electrical stimulation are also sometimes used to help relax the pelvic floor muscles. In some cases, surgery may be necessary to treat pelvic floor dysfunction. If you are suffering from pelvic floor dysfunction, it is important to talk to your doctor to find out what treatment options are best for you.

What triggers pelvic floor dysfunction?

The pelvic floor is a group of muscles and ligaments that support the pelvic organs, including the bladder, uterus, and bowel. Pelvic floor dysfunction (PFD) is a condition that can occur when these muscles and ligaments are weakened or damaged. This can lead to problems such as incontinence, prolapse, and pain during sex. There are a number of things that can trigger PFD, including: -Pregnancy and childbirth: The process of giving birth can damage the pelvic floor muscles and ligaments. This is especially true if you have a vaginal delivery. -Age: The pelvic floor muscles and ligaments can weaken with age. This is often due to the natural aging process, as well as the loss of estrogen that occurs after menopause. -Chronic cough: Frequent coughing can put a lot of strain on the pelvic floor muscles and ligaments. -Being overweight: Extra weight can put pressure on the pelvic floor muscles and ligaments. -Constipation: Straining to have a bowel movement can weaken the pelvic floor muscles and ligaments. -Anal intercourse: This can cause small tears in the lining of the anus, which can lead to PFD. If you think you may be experiencing PFD, it's important to see a doctor. There are a number of treatments that can help, including pelvic floor physical therapy, weight loss, and, in some cases, surgery.

What does pelvic floor pain feel like?

Pelvic floor pain can feel like a sharp pain, or a dull ache. It can be constant, or come and go. It can be felt in the vagina, vulva, anus, or lower back. The pain may get worse during sex, or when you put pressure on the pelvic floor muscles, like when you sneeze, cough, or sit for a long time. For some women, the pain is only a minor annoyance. But for others, it can be so severe that it interferes with their daily activities. If you have pelvic floor pain, it's important to talk to your doctor so they can help you find the cause and treat the pain.

Where do you feel pelvic floor dysfunction?

Pelvic floor dysfunction can present itself in a number of ways. The most common symptom is a feeling of heaviness or pressure in the pelvic region. This can be accompanied by pain in the lower back, hips, or thighs. Other symptoms include urinary or fecal incontinence, difficulty emptying the bladder or bowels, and pain during sex. pelvic floor dysfunction can be caused by a number of things, including pregnancy, childbirth, menopause, obesity, and chronic constipation. It can also be the result of injury to the pelvic floor muscles or nerves. There are a number of treatment options available for pelvic floor dysfunction. These include physical therapy, biofeedback, and electrical stimulation. Surgery is also an option, although it is usually only recommended as a last resort. If you are experiencing any of the symptoms of pelvic floor dysfunction, it is important to see your doctor so that the cause can be determined and appropriate treatment can be started.

The pelvic floor is a group of muscles, ligaments, and connective tissue that forms a bowl-shaped structure at the bottom of the pelvis. The pelvic floor supports the pelvic organs, including the bladder, uterus, and rectum, and maintains continence by closing the urethra and anal canal. The muscles of the pelvic floor can be weak or damaged by childbirth, pregnancy, surgery, and other conditions, which can lead to urinary and fecal incontinence. pelvic floor exercises, such as Kegels, can help to strengthen the muscles and improve continence.

Does pelvic floor dysfunction ever go away?

Pelvic floor dysfunction (PFD) is a condition that can cause a variety of symptoms, including pain in the pelvic area, difficulty urinating, or sexual dysfunction. While there is no cure for PFD, there are treatments that can improve symptoms. In many cases, PFD does not go away completely, but the symptoms can be managed to the point where they no longer significantly interfere with quality of life. The pelvic floor is a group of muscles and tissues that support the organs in the pelvis, including the bladder, uterus, and rectum. These muscles and tissues can become weak or damaged, causing problems with function. PFD can be caused by a variety of factors, including pregnancy, childbirth, menopause, obesity, or chronic constipation. There are a number of different treatments for PFD, depending on the underlying cause. If the cause is weakened muscles, pelvic floor muscle training (PFMT) can be effective. PFMT is a type of exercise that strengthens the pelvic floor muscles. It can be done at home, and often requires no special equipment. It is important to seek guidance from a pelvic floor physical therapist to ensure that the exercises are being done correctly. For those with PFD caused by damage to the pelvic floor tissues, treatments such as injectable fillers, laser therapy, or surgery may be recommended. These treatments can help to repair the damaged tissue and improve symptoms. In some cases, surgery may be the only option. PFD can be a chronic condition, but with proper treatment, symptoms can be managed and quality of life can be improved. In some cases, PFD may even go away completely. However, it is important to remember that PFD is a chronic condition, and there is a possibility that symptoms may return. Even with treatment, PFD can be a lifelong condition.

How do you test for pelvic floor dysfunction?

What is pelvic floor dysfunction? Pelvic floor dysfunction is a condition that can occur when the muscles and tissues that support the pelvic organs become weak or damaged. This can lead to problems with bowel and bladder control, sexual function, and pain in the pelvis. How do you test for pelvic floor dysfunction? There are a number of ways to test for pelvic floor dysfunction, including: Medical history and physical examination: Your doctor will ask about your symptoms and medical history, and will perform a physical examination. Pelvic floor muscle assessment: This involves testing the strength and function of the pelvic floor muscles. This can be done manually or with specialised equipment. Anorectal manometry: This test measures the pressure in the rectum and anal canal. A small, soft tube is inserted into the anus and the pressure is measured. Pelvic ultrasonography: This is a type of ultrasound that produces images of the pelvic organs and tissues. defecography: This is an X-ray test that is used to assess how well the rectum and anal sphincter are functioning. A soft, liquid contrast material is inserted into the rectum and X-rays are taken. MRI defecography: This is a type of MRI that produces images of the pelvic organs and tissues. A small amount of liquid contrast material is inserted into the rectum and images are taken. Your doctor will choose the best tests for you based on your symptoms and medical history.

Can you reverse pelvic floor dysfunction?

Pelvic floor dysfunction (PFD) is a condition that can affect both men and women, although it is more common in women. PFD can cause a number of problems, including urinary incontinence, fecal incontinence, and sexual dysfunction. Most cases of PFD can be successfully treated, often with a combination of lifestyle changes, physical therapy, and medication. In some cases, surgery may be necessary. There is no single answer to the question of whether or not PFD can be reversed. The answer depends on the individual case, the severity of the PFD, and the underlying cause. In many cases, PFD can be controlled and even reversed with lifestyle changes and physical therapy. For example, Kegel exercises can strengthen the pelvic floor muscles and help to treat urinary incontinence. In some cases, surgery may be necessary to correct the underlying problem, such as a prolapsed uterus or rectocele. However, even in these cases, lifestyle changes and physical therapy can often help to improve the condition. PFD is a condition that can be debilitating and cause a great deal of distress. However, in most cases, it can be effectively treated. If you are experiencing any of the symptoms associated with PFD, talk to your doctor to discuss your treatment options.

What to avoid with pelvic floor dysfunction?

As someone with pelvic floor dysfunction, there are certain activities and lifestyle choices that can make your symptoms worse. Here are some things to avoid if you have pelvic floor dysfunction: -Lifting heavy objects: Any type of lifting can put strain on the pelvic floor muscles and cause them to spasm or tighten. This is why activities like weight-lifting or even picking up a child can be difficult for people with pelvic floor dysfunction. -Sitting for long periods of time: This can put pressure on the pelvic floor muscles and cause them to fatigue. Try to take breaks often to stand up and move around. -Wearing tight clothing: clothing that is tight around the waist or groin can put pressure on the pelvic floor muscles and aggravate symptoms. Try to wear loose-fitting clothes and avoid anything that constricts the area. -Doing high-impact activities: activities like running or jumping can jar the pelvic floor and cause pain. If you enjoy these activities, try to do them on softer surfaces like a treadmill or an exercise mat. -Having constipation: this can worsen pelvic floor dysfunction symptoms like pain and spasms. Eat a high-fiber diet and drink plenty of fluids to avoid constipation. -Avoiding exercise: While it may be tempting to rest and avoid activities that make your symptoms worse, it's important to keep the pelvic floor muscles strong. Try to find low-impact exercises that don't aggravate your symptoms and talk to your doctor before starting any new exercise routine.

How common is pelvic floor dysfunction?

It's estimated that about one in every three women will experience some form of pelvic floor dysfunction in their lifetime. So, while it's certainly not an uncommon problem, it's one that many women suffer from in silence. There are a number of reasons why pelvic floor dysfunction can be such a taboo subject. For one, it can be seen as a very personal issue and many women feel embarrassed or ashamed to talk about it. Additionally, the symptoms of pelvic floor dysfunction can be both physically and emotionally extremely painful and can have a significant impact on a woman's quality of life. Pelvic floor dysfunction can cause a range of symptoms, including pain during sex, pain when urinating or defecating, incontinence, and a feeling of heaviness or pressure in the pelvis. These symptoms can have a profound impact on a woman's ability to enjoy sex, to work, or to perform everyday activities. While pelvic floor dysfunction can be a very difficult and debilitating problem, there are treatments available that can help. Physical therapy and specific exercises are often successful in alleviating symptoms and restoring quality of life. Surgery is also an option for some women, depending on the severity of their symptoms. If you're experiencing any of the above symptoms, don't suffer in silence. Talk to your doctor about pelvic floor dysfunction and ask about the treatment options that are available to you.

How long does it take to fix weak pelvic floor?

It's estimated that approximately one in three women in the United States experience some form of pelvic floor dysfunction. The most common symptom of weak pelvic floor muscles is urine leakage, which can range from a small dribble to severe incontinence. Other symptoms include pelvic pain, difficulty emptying your bladder or bowels, and a feeling of heaviness or pressure in your pelvic region. So, how long does it take to fix weak pelvic floor muscles? The truth is, there is no one-size-fits-all answer to this question. The amount of time it will take to see results depends on a number of individual factors, including the severity of your symptoms, the underlying cause of your pelvic floor dysfunction, and your overall health. That being said, most women who commit to a pelvic floor strengthening program see significant improvement within 12 weeks. For some women, the results are even more dramatic, with a significant reduction in symptoms after just a few weeks of regular pelvic floor exercises. If you are suffering from symptoms of weak pelvic floor muscles, the best thing you can do is talk to your doctor. They will be able to give you a more specific timeline for how long it will take to see results based on your individual situation. In the meantime, start practicing some of the pelvic floor strengthening exercises that are most effective for treating pelvic floor dysfunction. With commitment and consistency, you will soon be on your way to a stronger, healthier pelvic floor.

Is walking good for tight pelvic floor?

Walking is a great way to help keep your pelvic floor healthy and strong. When you walk, your pelvic floor muscles work to keep your pelvis stable. This helps to tone the muscles and keep them strong. Additionally, walking can help to prevent constipation, which can also help to keep your pelvic floor healthy. There are a few things to keep in mind when you are walking for your pelvic floor. First, make sure to wear comfortable shoes. This will help to avoid any strain on your feet, ankles, or legs. Second, walking at a moderate pace is ideal. You don't want to overdo it and put too much strain on your body. Finally, be sure to listen to your body. If you start to feel pain or discomfort, stop and rest. Overall, walking is a great way to help keep your pelvic floor healthy and strong. by keeping your muscles toned and preventing constipation. Just be sure to walk at a moderate pace and listen to your body if you start to feel any discomfort.

The pelvic floor is a group of muscles and ligaments that support the bladder, uterus, and rectum. These muscles and ligaments can be weakened by pregnancy, childbirth, surgery, and aging. This can lead to urinary incontinence, pelvic organ prolapse, and sexual dysfunction. There are many treatments available to strengthen the pelvic floor, including exercises, weights, and electrical stimulation.

How painful can pelvic floor dysfunction be?

Pelvic floor dysfunction can be extremely painful. The pelvic floor is a group of muscles and tissues that support the bladder, uterus, and rectum. These muscles and tissues can become weak or tight, which can cause pain in the pelvic region. The pain can range from a dull ache to a sharp pain. For some women, the pain is so severe that it interferes with their daily activities. There are several treatments available for pelvic floor dysfunction. Physical therapy is often recommended to help strengthen the pelvic floor muscles. Medications, such as muscle relaxants, can also be prescribed to help relieve the pain. In some cases, surgery may be necessary to correct the problem. If you are experiencing pain in the pelvic region, it is important to see your doctor. He or she can determine the cause of the pain and recommend the best treatment for you.

What medication is used for pelvic floor dysfunction?

There are a few different types of medication that can be used to help treat pelvic floor dysfunction. The first type is medication that helps to relax the muscles in the pelvic floor. This can be helpful in relieving some of the symptoms of pelvic floor dysfunction, such as pain and muscle spasms. The second type of medication that can be used is medication that helps to increase the strength of the muscles in the pelvic floor. This can be helpful in treating the cause of pelvic floor dysfunction, which is often weak or damaged muscles. The third type of medication that can be used is medication that helps to improve the function of the nerves in the pelvic floor. This can be helpful in treating the symptoms of pelvic floor dysfunction, such as pain, numbness, and tingling.

What exercises weaken pelvic floor?

There are a number of exercises that can weaken the pelvic floor. These include activities such as sit-ups, leg lifts, or any type of activity that puts strain on the abdomen. Other exercises that can weaken the pelvic floor include coughing, sneezing, and even laughing. These activities all put strain on the pelvic floor muscles and can lead to weakened muscles and eventual incontinence. If you are concerned about weakening your pelvic floor, it is important to talk to your doctor or a qualified physical therapist to learn about which exercises are safe for you to do.

Can stress and anxiety cause pelvic floor dysfunction?

It's well known that stress and anxiety can lead to all sorts of physical health problems. But can these mental health issues also cause pelvic floor dysfunction? The pelvic floor is a group of muscles and tissues that support the bladder, uterus, and rectum. When these muscles are weak or become damaged, it can lead to problems such as incontinence, discomfort during sex, and pain in the lower abdomen. There are a number of things that can cause pelvic floor dysfunction, including childbirth, surgery, and certain types of medications. But stress and anxiety can also play a role. For many people, stress and anxiety lead to changes in their bathroom habits. They may start to urinate more often, or they may develop diarrhea or constipation. These changes can put extra strain on the pelvic floor muscles, leading to weakness and damage. In addition, when we're feeling stressed or anxious, we tend to hold our breath or hold in our stomach muscles. This can also lead to pelvic floor problems, as it can cause the muscles to become overstretched or to spasm. If you're dealing with stress or anxiety, it's important to find healthy ways to cope. This may include exercise, relaxation techniques, and talking to a therapist. If you're also dealing with pelvic floor dysfunction, there are treatments that can help, including physical therapy and medications. Don't hesitate to talk to your doctor about what's going on and what options are available to you.

Does drinking water help with pelvic floor?

It is a common misconception that drinking water will help to 'flush out' any pelvic floor problems. The pelvic floor is a group of muscles, ligaments and tissues that support the bladder, bowel and uterus. These muscles can be weakened or damaged due to pregnancy, childbirth, surgery, being overweight, chronic coughing or constipation. While drinking water can help to prevent some of these issues, it will not always help to alleviate symptoms or improve muscle function. There are many things that can contribute to pelvic floor problems, and each person may experience different symptoms. For some, Pelvic floor exercises may be enough to strengthen the muscles and improve function. Others may need to seek medical help, as their pelvic floor dysfunction may be caused by an underlying medical condition. If you are experiencing any problems with your pelvic floor, it is important to see a doctor or other healthcare professional to rule out any serious causes. Once a diagnosis has been made, they can advise on the best course of treatment. This may include Pelvic floor exercises, medication, or surgery.

What age does pelvic floor dysfunction occur?

Pelvic floor dysfunction occurs when the muscles and tissues that support the pelvis weaken or are injured. This can happen at any age, but is more common in older adults. Pelvic floor muscles help to control the bowel and bladder, and to support the pelvis and organs. When these muscles are weak or damaged, they can't do their job properly. This can lead to problems such as incontinence (leakage of urine or stool), prolapse (organs falling down into the vagina), and pain during sex. There are many things that can contribute to pelvic floor dysfunction, including childbirth, pregnancy, aging, chronic constipation or diarrhea, and being overweight. Often, there is no single cause, and the condition may develop over time. If you are experiencing any of the symptoms of pelvic floor dysfunction, talk to your doctor. There are many things that can be done to help, including exercises to strengthen the muscles, diet and lifestyle changes, and in some cases, medication or surgery.

What does pelvic floor physiotherapy include?

Pelvic floor physiotherapy is a type of physical therapy that helps to strengthen and improve the function of the pelvic floor muscles. These muscles support the pelvic organs,including the bladder and uterus, and help to control urinary and fecal incontinence. Pelvic floor physiotherapy can help to improve the function of the pelvic floor muscles and reduce urinary and fecal incontinence. The physiotherapist will assess the muscle strength and function and prescribe exercises to improve the muscle tone. They will also teach the correct techniques for performing the exercises. The physiotherapist may also recommend other treatments, such as electrical stimulation or biofeedback, to help improve the function of the pelvic floor muscles.

There is still much unknown about the pelvic floor, but what is known is that it is an essential part of the female body. It supports the uterus and bowel, and helps to control the passage of urine and feces. Additionally, the pelvic floor muscles help to sexual function and orgasm. Because of its vital role, it is important to keep the pelvic floor healthy through exercise and proper nutrition.

What is the best sleeping position for pelvic floor?

The best sleeping position for the pelvic floor is on the back with a pillow under the knees. This position takes the pressure off of the pelvic floor and allows for the muscles to relax. Sleeping on the side or stomach can put pressure on the pelvic floor and cause the muscles to become tense.

What is the best sleeping position to relax pelvic floor?

There are several sleeping positions that can help relax the pelvic floor. One is sleeping on your back with a pillow under your knees. This position takes the pressure off the pelvic floor and can help to ease any pain or discomfort. Another position is sleeping on your side with a pillow between your legs. This position also takes the pressure off the pelvic floor and can help to reduce any pain or discomfort. Lastly, sleeping on your stomach with a pillow under your hips can also help to take the pressure off the pelvic floor and can ease any pain or discomfort. Whichever position you choose, make sure that you are comfortable and that your pelvis is in a neutral position.

What position should I sleep in for pelvic pain?

There are a few different positions that you can sleep in if you're experiencing pelvic pain. One position is to sleep on your back with a pillow under your knees. This position takes the pressure off of your lower back and pelvis. Another position is to sleep on your side with a pillow between your legs. This position also takes the pressure off of your lower back and pelvis. Lastly, you can sleep on your stomach with a pillow under your hips. This position can help relieve pain by taking the pressure off of your pelvis and lower back. The best position to sleep in for pelvic pain will vary from person to person. It is important to experiment with different positions to find the one that is most comfortable for you. If you find that you are still experiencing pain in a certain position, you may want to try another position. Sleeping in a comfortable position can help you get a good night's sleep, which can in turn help you deal with pelvic pain during the day.

Can pelvic floor dysfunction happen suddenly?

Pelvic floor dysfunction can happen suddenly in some cases, although it is more likely to develop gradually over time. The pelvic floor is a group of muscles and tissues that support the pelvic organs, including the bladder, uterus, and rectum. These muscles and tissues can become weak or damaged, which can lead to urinary or fecal incontinence, pelvic pain, or sexual dysfunction. There are several factors that can contribute to the development of pelvic floor dysfunction, including childbirth, surgery, menopause, and aging. Childbirth is the most common cause of pelvic floor dysfunction, as the process of delivering a baby can weaken or damage the muscles and tissues of the pelvic floor. Surgery, particularly abdominal or pelvic surgery, can also cause pelvic floor dysfunction. Menopause can contribute to the development of pelvic floor dysfunction because the loss of estrogen can lead to the thinning and weakening of the pelvic floor muscles and tissues. Aging can also lead to the development of pelvic floor dysfunction, as the aging process can cause the muscles and tissues of the pelvic floor to weaken and deteriorate. There are several treatment options available for pelvic floor dysfunction, including pelvic floor muscle exercises, electrical stimulation, and surgery. Pelvic floor muscle exercises, also known as Kegel exercises, can help to strengthen the muscles and tissues of the pelvic floor. Electrical stimulation can help to improve muscle function and reduce pain. Surgery can be used to repair damaged muscles and tissues, or to remove excess tissue. Pelvic floor dysfunction can be a difficult condition to deal with, but there are treatment options available that can help to improve symptoms. If you think you may be dealing with pelvic floor dysfunction, it is important to talk to your doctor so that you can get the appropriate treatment.

Does pelvic floor dysfunction make you tired?

There are a lot of things that can contribute to fatigue, and pelvic floor dysfunction is one of them. When your pelvic floor muscles are weak or not functioning properly, it can lead to a feeling of fatigue. There are a number of factors that can contribute to pelvic floor dysfunction, including pregnancy, childbirth, menopause, and constipation. Pregnancy is one of the most common causes of pelvic floor dysfunction. The added weight of the baby can put a strain on the muscles and ligaments in the pelvis, which can lead to weakness and dysfunction. Childbirth can also cause pelvic floor dysfunction. The process of pushing the baby out can cause the muscles and ligaments to stretch and tear, which can lead to weakness and dysfunction. Menopause can also cause pelvic floor dysfunction. As women go through menopause, they can experience a loss of estrogen, which can lead to thinning of the pelvic floor muscles and ligaments. This can cause the muscles to weaken and not function properly. Constipation can also cause pelvic floor dysfunction. When you are constipated, you may strain to have a bowel movement. This can put a strain on the muscles and ligaments in the pelvis, which can lead to weakness and dysfunction. Pelvic floor dysfunction can cause a feeling of fatigue. There are a number of things that can contribute to pelvic floor dysfunction, including pregnancy, childbirth, menopause, and constipation. If you are experiencing fatigue, it is important to talk to your doctor to find out if pelvic floor dysfunction may be the cause.

Can pelvic floor dysfunction be hormonal?

The pelvic floor is a group of muscles, ligaments, and connective tissue that supports the bladder, uterus, and rectum. It also helps to control bowel and bladder function. Pelvic floor dysfunction (PFD) is when the pelvic floor muscles and ligaments are not working properly. This can cause problems with urination, bowel movements, and sexual function. PFD can be caused by a variety of things, including pregnancy, childbirth, surgery, aging, and chronic conditions such as constipation or diarrhea. There is a lot of debate about whether or not PFD can be caused by hormones. Some experts say that PFD is not caused by hormones, but by other factors such as pregnancy or aging. Other experts say that hormones can play a role in PFD. It is hard to say for sure if hormones are a cause of PFD because there is not enough research on the topic. Some studies have found a link between PFD and hormone levels, but more research is needed to confirm these results. If you are experiencing PFD, talk to your doctor about possible causes and treatment options.

What is the best vitamin for pelvic floor?

There are a lot of things that can contribute to poor pelvic floor health, including pregnancy, childbirth, being overweight, and chronic coughing or constipation. Because of this, there isn't just one "best" vitamin for pelvic floor health. Instead, there are several vitamins and minerals that can help to support a healthy pelvic floor. Some good options for vitamins and minerals that support the pelvic floor include calcium, vitamin D, and magnesium. Calcium is essential for bone health, and vitamin D helps the body to absorb calcium. Magnesium is also important for bone health, and it can also help to relax muscles. Another important vitamin for the pelvic floor is vitamin C. Vitamin C is a powerful antioxidants and it helps to support the health of connective tissue. This is important because the pelvic floor is made up of connective tissue, and this tissue can be damaged by things like inflammation. Some other vitamins and minerals that may be helpful for the pelvic floor include vitamin E, B-complex vitamins, and zinc. Vitamin E is another powerful antioxidant, and it can help to protect the body from damage caused by free radicals. B-complex vitamins are important for the health of the nervous system, and zinc is essential for wound healing. While there are many different vitamins and minerals that can support the health of the pelvic floor, it's important to talk to your doctor or midwife before taking any supplements. This is because some supplements can interact with medications, and some of them are not safe for pregnant or breastfeeding women. If you're looking for ways to support your pelvic floor health, there are also some lifestyle changes you can make. For example, you can try to maintain a healthy weight, and you can avoid smoking and excessive alcohol consumption. You can also try to do exercises that focus on strengthening the pelvic floor muscles, such as Kegel exercises.

Pelvic floor exercises are a great way to improve your overall health and well-being. By strengthening your pelvic floor muscles, you can improve your bladder and bowel control, sexual function, and reduce your risk of injuries during exercise and activities.

What supplements help tight pelvic floor?

In order to maintain a tight pelvic floor, it is important to keep the muscles strong and healthy. There are a few different supplements that can help to achieve this. One supplement that can be beneficial for the pelvic floor is magnesium. This mineral is involved in muscle contraction and relaxation, and can help to keep the pelvic floor muscles healthy and strong. It can also help to reduce stress and anxiety, which can contribute to tension in the pelvic floor muscles. Another supplement that can help to support the pelvic floor is vitamin D. This vitamin is necessary for calcium absorption, and can help to keep the pelvic floor muscles strong and healthy. It is also involved in immune function, and can help to reduce the risk of infection in the pelvic area. Fish oil supplements are also a good option for supporting the pelvic floor. Fish oil is a good source of omega-3 fatty acids, which are known for their anti-inflammatory properties. Inflammation can contribute to tension in the pelvic floor muscles, so keeping inflammation under control can help to reduce pelvic floor pain and discomfort.

Finally, probiotics can also be beneficial for the pelvic floor. Probiotics help to maintain a healthy balance of bacteria in the gut, and can help to reduce the risk of infection in the pelvic area. They can also help to reduce inflammation and support immune function.

Do you have to undress for pelvic floor therapy?

Do you have to undress for pelvic floor therapy? It depends. Sometimes, your therapist may need to see your pelvic area to properly assess and treat your condition. In these cases, you will likely need to undress. However, if your therapist is only working on your back or legs, you will probably not need to undress. If you do need to undress, you will be given a gown or sheet to cover yourself with. You will always be given the option to keep your underwear on if you feel more comfortable. Your therapist will never force you to do anything you are not comfortable with. If you have any concerns about undressing for therapy, please talk to your therapist. They will be more than happy to answer any questions or concerns you may have.

Do I need to shave for pelvic floor physical therapy?

There is no right or wrong answer to whether or not you should shave for pelvic floor physical therapy. It is ultimately up to you and what you are comfortable with. If you are comfortable with it, shaving may help the physical therapist get a better view and understanding of your pelvic floor muscles. It may also help the physical therapist to better target the muscles that need to be worked on. However, if you are not comfortable with shaving, that is perfectly okay too. There are other ways that the physical therapist can assess your pelvic floor muscles. For example, they may use a mirror or ask you to do a self-assessment. Ultimately, the decision of whether or not to shave for your pelvic floor physical therapy appointment is up to you. If you have any questions or concerns, be sure to discuss them with your physical therapist beforehand.

What is a pelvic floor massage?

There are many benefits that come with getting a pelvic floor massage. For one, it can help to release any tightness or tension that may be present in the pelvic floor muscles. This can lead to an overall sense of wellbeing and relaxation. The massage can also help to increase blood circulation in the area, which can promote healing. In addition, a pelvic floor massage can also be helpful in treating or preventing problems with incontinence. When the muscles of the pelvic floor are weak, it can lead to a loss of control over the bladder or bowel. This can be a very embarrassing and frustrating problem. A pelvic floor massage can help to strengthen the muscles, which can lead to better control and fewer accidents. If you are considering getting a pelvic floor massage, it is important to find a qualified therapist who has experience in this type of massage. It is also important to communicate with your therapist about any discomfort or pain you may be experiencing. This type of massage should not be painful, but if it is, it is important to let your therapist know so they can adjust their technique.

Is pelvic floor physical therapy embarrassing?

For many people, the thought of pelvic floor physical therapy (PT) is embarrassing. It can be tough to face the reality that something may be wrong down there, and even tougher to imagine discussing it with a stranger. But here's the thing: pelvic floor PT is nothing to be embarrassed about. In fact, it's a very common issue, and one that affects people of all ages and genders. The pelvic floor is a group of muscles and tissues that support the bladder, uterus, and rectum. These muscles can be weakened by pregnancy, childbirth, surgery, and age. When they're weak, they can't do their job properly, which can lead to incontinence, pain, and other issues. Pelvic floor PT can help to strengthen these muscles and improve function. The treatments are usually painless and non-invasive, and can be done in the privacy of your own home. If you're experiencing any symptoms that could be related to a weak pelvic floor, don't hesitate to reach out to a PT. There's no need to be embarrassed—they've heard it all before, and they're there to help.

How do you fix pelvic organ prolapse?

When you hear the term "pelvic floor," you may not be entirely sure what it is. Your pelvic floor is a group of muscles, ligaments and tissues that form a bowl-like structure at the base of your pelvis. These muscles and tissues support your bladder, uterus and rectum. If you have pelvic organ prolapse, it means that one or more of these organs has fallen out of place and is pressing against the walls of your vagina. pelvic organ prolapse can be caused by a number of things, including pregnancy, childbirth, obesity and repetitive heavy lifting. There are a number of ways to treat pelvic organ prolapse, depending on the severity of your prolapse and the organs involved. If your prolapse is mild, you may be able to treat it with lifestyle changes, such as losing weight, avoiding constipation and avoiding activities that put strain on your pelvic floor. If your prolapse is more severe, you may need to have surgery to fix it. Surgery options include vaginal prolapse surgery, uterine prolapse surgery and sacrocolpopexy. Vaginal prolapse surgery involves placing supports in your vagina to hold your organs in place. Uterine prolapse surgery involves stitching your uterus in place so that it doesn't fall out of your vagina. Sacrocolpopexy is a type of surgery that involves attaching your pelvic organs to your sacrum, which is the bone at the base of your spine. No matter what treatment option you choose, it's important to see your doctor if you think you have pelvic organ prolapse. prolapse can cause problems with urinating and having a bowel movement, as well as pain during sex. If you don't treat your prolapse, it can lead to more serious problems, such as urinary incontinence and kidney damage.

How serious is pelvic organ prolapse?

Pelvic organ prolapse is a condition in which one or more of the pelvic organs drops down from its original position and into the vaginal canal. The most common organs affected are the bladder, the uterus, and the rectum. While most cases of pelvic organ prolapse are not serious, some can lead to urinary incontinence and difficulty emptying the bladder. In severe cases, the prolapsed organ may protrude from the vagina. If you are experiencing any symptoms of pelvic organ prolapse, it is important to see a doctor to determine the severity of the condition. Treatment options vary depending on the severity of the prolapse, but may include pelvic floor exercises, vaginal pessaries, or surgery.

The pelvic floor is an important part of the female anatomy. It supports the uterus and other organs, and helps to control the flow of urine. Pelvic floor dysfunction can cause incontinence, pelvic pain, and sexual dysfunction. Treatment of pelvic floor dysfunction can be difficult, but there are many options available.

What is the most common cause of pelvic organ prolapse?

Pelvic organ prolapse is a condition in which one or more of the organs in the pelvis slip down from their normal position and protrude into the vaginal canal. The most common type of prolapse is when the uterus (womb) slips down into the vaginal canal. This is known as uterine prolapse. Other types of prolapse include: - when the top of the vagina slips down into the vaginal canal (vaginal prolapse) - when the bowel slips down into the vaginal canal (rectocele) - when the bladder slips down into the vaginal canal (cystocele or bladder prolapse) The most common cause of pelvic organ prolapse is a weakening of the tissues and muscles that support the organs in the pelvis. This can happen for a number of reasons, including: - childbirth - prorates - menopause - being overweight or obese - chronic cough or constipation Pelvic organ prolapse is a very common condition, particularly in women who have had children. It is estimated that 1 in 3 women will experience some form of prolapse in their lifetime. While it is most common in older women, it can occur at any age.

How do I check myself for pelvic organ prolapse?

There are several ways to check for pelvic organ prolapse. The most common is the pelvic organ prolapse quantification (POP-Q) system, which uses points to measure the descent of the pelvic organs. The POP-Q system is followed by a pelvic examination, during which the doctor checks for tissue protruding from the vaginal opening. Another way to check for pelvic organ prolapse is to use an ultrasound. This is usually done when the doctor suspects that there is a prolapse but the POP-Q system does not confirm it. Ultrasound can also be used to measure the size of the prolapse. The third way to check for pelvic organ prolapse is to use MRI. This is the most expensive and least common method, but it is the most accurate.

Can I push my pelvic prolapse back up?

When you have a pelvic prolapse, it can feel like you are constantly on the verge of losing control of your bladder or bowels. This can be a very scary and embarrassing feeling. Many people with a pelvic prolapse wonder if they will ever be able to control their bladder or bowels again. The good news is that, in most cases, a pelvic prolapse is not a permanent condition. With proper treatment and care, most people with a pelvic prolapse will be able to control their bladder and bowels and live a normal, healthy life. There are several treatment options for a pelvic prolapse. The best option for you will depend on the severity of your prolapse and your overall health. In some cases, a simple lifestyle change, such as losing weight or avoiding constipation, may be enough to relieve your symptoms. Other times, you may need surgery to repair the prolapse. If your prolapse is mild, your doctor may recommend that you try a pelvic floor muscle training program. This type of program can help to strengthen the muscles that support the pelvic organs and may help to reduce the symptoms of a prolapse. In some cases, a pelvic prolapse can be pushed back into place. This is called a reduction. A reduction may be done in the doctor's office or in the hospital. In most cases, a reduction is only done if the prolapse is small and does not cause pain or other symptoms. If your prolapse is more severe, you may need surgery to repair it. Surgery can be done to repair the uterine prolapse, rectal prolapse, or vaginal prolapse. The type of surgery that you have will depend on the type of prolapse that you have and your overall health. After surgery, you will likely need to stay in the hospital for a few days. You may also need to take pain medication and have someone help you with activities of daily living for a short time. Most people are able to return to their normal activities within a few weeks. If you have a pelvic prolapse, it is important to talk to your doctor about your treatment options. With proper treatment, most people with a pelvic prolapse will be able to control their symptoms and live a normal, healthy life.

Can you push a prolapse back into place?

A prolapse is a condition where organs in the pelvis slip down from their original position. The most common type of prolapse is a vaginal prolapse, which occurs when the uterus, cervix, or bladder protrudes through the vaginal opening. While a prolapse cannot be cured, there are treatments available to help ease symptoms and keep the prolapse from getting worse.

One common question women with a prolapse ask is whether or not they can push the prolapse back into place. While it is possible to push a prolapse back into place, it is not recommended. Doing so can cause further damage to the already weakened pelvic floor muscles and surrounding tissue. Additionally, many women find that the prolapse pops back out soon after they try to push it back in. If you are struggling with a prolapse, it is best to talk to your doctor or a pelvic floor specialist to find the best treatment option for you.

What happens if you don't fix a prolapse?

If you have a prolapse, it means that one or more of your pelvic organs has fallen out of place. Usually, this means that your uterus has descended into your vagina. A prolapse can happen when the muscles and ligaments that support your pelvic organs weaken or loosen. Prolapses are common—they affect about one in three women at some point in their lives. They can happen to women of any age, but are more common after menopause. Most prolapses are not harmful, but they can cause pain and other problems. If left untreated, a prolapse can get worse over time. In severe cases, it can lead to incontinence (leakage of urine or feces). If you have a prolapse, there are several things you can do to treat it. These include: · Wearing a special support garment, such as a pessary or a vaginal support device · Doing pelvic floor exercises to strengthen the muscles that support your pelvic organs · Taking medication to help with pain or incontinence · Having surgery to repair the prolapse If you have a prolapse, it is important to see your doctor so that you can discuss your treatment options.

At what age does pelvic organ prolapse occur?

Pelvic organ prolapse occurs when the pelvic organs — the bladder, uterus, and rectum — drop from their normal position and press against the wall of the vagina. This can happen at any age, but it is most common after menopause. At least one in four women over the age of 50 will develop prolapse of the bladder or uterus. Most cases of pelvic organ prolapse are caused by a combination of factors. The most important factor is pregnancy and childbirth. The more pregnancies a woman has, the greater her likelihood of developing prolapse. Other factors that may contribute to prolapse include: -Being overweight or obese -Chronic coughing -Constipation -Frequent heavy lifting -Genetics -Menopause -Smoking If you have any of these risk factors, you should talk to your doctor about ways to reduce your risk of developing prolapse.

How do you know if your pelvic floor has dropped?

The pelvic floor is a group of muscles and ligaments that support the bladder, uterus, and rectum. These muscles and ligaments can be weakened by pregnancy, childbirth, age, or weight gain. When the pelvic floor is weakened, it can cause the organs it supports to drop, or prolapse. There are several signs that can indicate that the pelvic floor has dropped. One sign is leaking urine when coughing, sneezing, or laughing. This happens because the muscles that normally support the urethra are not as strong, and the urethra cannot close properly. Leaking feces or difficulty controlling bowel movements is another sign of a weak pelvic floor. This can happen when the rectum prolapses, or drops down, into the vagina. prolapse. Pain in the pelvic area is another symptom. This pain can be caused by the prolapse of the uterus, bladder, or rectum into the vagina. If you are experiencing any of these symptoms, it is important to talk to your doctor. They can perform a pelvic exam to determine if your pelvic floor has dropped.

There are a number of things that can be done to keep the pelvic floor healthy and strong. Regular exercise, especially core-strengthening activities, can help to prevent problems with the pelvic floor. If you are already experiencing problems with the pelvic floor, there are a number of treatments that can help, including physical therapy and medications.

Can you naturally fix a pelvic prolapse?

A pelvic prolapse is a condition in which one or more of the pelvic organs (bladder, uterus, rectum, or vagina) falls down into or out of the vagina. Pelvic prolapse is often caused by pregnancy and childbirth, but it can also be caused by obesity, menopause, and certain medical conditions. There is no one-size-fits-all answer to the question of whether or not a pelvic prolapse can be naturally fixed. In some cases, a pelvic prolapse may resolve itself without any treatment, but in other cases, medical intervention may be necessary. For example, if the prolapse is severe or if it is causing pain or other symptoms, surgery may be the best option. Pelvic prolapse is a serious condition that can cause a great deal of discomfort and inconvenience. If you are experiencing any symptoms of pelvic prolapse, it is important to see a doctor so that you can get the treatment you need.

Will walking make prolapse worse?

Prolapse is a condition that can happen when the organs in your pelvis slip out of place. This can happen if the muscles and ligaments that hold everything in place become weak. If you have prolapse, you might notice a bulge in your vagina. This can happen when you stand for a long time, cough, or strain during a bowel movement. Walking is a great exercise for your overall health, but it is not recommended if you have prolapse. This is because when you walk, your abdominal muscles contract and put pressure on your pelvic floor. This can cause the organs in your pelvis to slip out of place even more. If you have prolapse, talking to your doctor about the best exercises for you.

Can you fix a pelvic prolapse without surgery?

A pelvic prolapse is a condition in which the pelvic organs—the bladder, uterus, or rectum—sag into the vaginal canal. In some cases, the prolapse may be only mild, causing no symptoms. In other cases, the prolapse may be more severe, resulting in urinary incontinence, difficulty urinating, or difficulty having a bowel movement. There are several possible causes of pelvic prolapse, including pregnancy, childbirth, menopause, and previous surgeries. Often, a combination of factors contributes to the condition. Pelvic prolapse is generally treated with surgery, which can be done vaginally or abdominally. In some cases, a prolapse can be treated without surgery, depending on the severity of the prolapse and the individual's symptoms. Non-surgical treatment options for pelvic prolapse include: - Supportive devices: A pessary is a device that is inserted into the vagina to support the pelvic organs and reduce prolapse symptoms. A pessary can be temporary or permanent. - Pelvic floor exercises: These exercises strengthen the muscles of the pelvic floor and can help to reduce prolapse symptoms. - Diet and lifestyle changes: Maintaining a healthy weight through diet and exercise can help to reduce the risk of pelvic prolapse. avoiding constipation can also help, as constipation can contribute to prolapse symptoms. If you are experiencing symptoms of pelvic prolapse, it is important to talk to your doctor. They will be able to discuss your treatment options with you and help you to make the best decision for your individual case.

How common is vaginal prolapse?

Vaginal prolapse is a condition that can occur when the pelvic floor muscles and ligaments weaken or loosen. This can cause the vagina or other organs, such as the bladder, to sag or drop down into the vaginal canal or out through the vaginal opening. Vaginal prolapse is a common condition, affecting about 50% of women over the age of 50.1 However, it can occur at any age.2 It is more common in women who have had one or more vaginal deliveries,3 but it can also occur in women who have never given birth.4 There are several types of vaginal prolapse, depending on which organs are affected. The most common type is anterior prolapse, which is when the front wall of the vagina drops down. Posterior prolapse, on the other hand, is when the back wall of the vagina drops down.5 Prolapse can also affect the urethra (the tube that carries urine from the bladder to the outside of the body), which is known as urethral prolapse.6 The symptoms of vaginal prolapse vary depending on the type and severity of the prolapse. In some cases, there may be no symptoms at all.7 However, the most common symptom is vaginal bulging or protrusion.8 This can be accompanied by pelvic pressure or discomfort, urinary incontinence, difficulty having a bowel movement, and/or painful intercourse.9 Vaginal prolapse is usually diagnosed through a physical exam, during which your doctor will check for signs of prolapse. They may also use a speculum to get a better view of the inside of the vagina.10 In some cases, further testing, such as an MRI or CT scan, may be needed to confirm the diagnosis. Treatment for vaginal prolapse often begins with lifestyle changes and/or pelvic floor exercises.11 If these interventions are not effective, surgery may be recommended. The type of surgery will depend on the type and severity of prolapse. For example, a pessary is a device that can be inserted into the vagina to support the organs and tissues.12 Surgery to correct prolapse may also involve stitching the tissues back into place or removing excess tissue.13 If you think you may be experiencing symptoms of vaginal prolapse, it is important to see your doctor. They can help you determine the cause of your symptoms and recommend the most effective treatment for you.

What does vaginal prolapse feel like?

Vaginal prolapse is a very common condition that can occur when the pelvic floor muscles weaken or are stretched. Prolapse occurs when the vaginal walls bulge or sag into the vaginal canal or outside of the vagina. While prolapse can happen to anyone, it is most common in women who have had children, are menopausal, or are obese. Most women with vaginal prolapse do not experience any pain or discomfort, but some may notice a bulge or lump in their vagina. Others may feel pressure in their pelvis or a sense of fullness in their vagina. In severe cases, women may have difficulty urinating or having a bowel movement. If you are experiencing any symptoms of vaginal prolapse, it is important to see your doctor. They will be able to diagnose the severity of your prolapse and recommend the best treatment options for you. In some cases, vaginal prolapse can be treated with pelvic floor exercises or a pessary, which is a small device that is inserted into the vagina to support the prolapsing organs. In other cases, surgery may be necessary to correct the prolapse.

Can you feel a uterine prolapse with your finger?

The pelvic floor is a group of muscles and ligaments that support the bladder, uterus, and rectum. The pelvic floor muscles surround the openings to the urethra, vagina, and anus. You cannot feel a uterine prolapse with your finger because the pelvic floor muscles and ligaments support the uterus and keep it in place. However, you may be able to feel a bulge in the vagina when the uterus prolapses.

Is walking good for prolapse?

The pelvic floor is a group of muscles and ligaments that supports the bladder, uterus, and bowel. These muscles and ligaments can be weakened by pregnancy, childbirth, age, and heavy lifting. A prolapse occurs when organs drop down from their normal position in the pelvis. Walking is a low-impact activity that can help to strengthen the muscles and ligaments of the pelvic floor. It is also a good way to get some exercise if you are pregnant or have recently given birth. Walking can help to prevent prolapse and can also help to reduce the symptoms of prolapse.

It's important to keep your pelvic floor strong and healthy! There are many ways to do this, including exercise, diet, and avoiding constipation. With a little effort, you can keep your pelvic floor functioning properly for years to come.

Can a tampon help prolapse?

A tampon can help prolapse in a couple ways. First, when you insert a tampon, it puts gentle pressure on the vaginal walls and the pelvic floor muscles. This pressure can help support the pelvic organs and prevent them from prolapsing. Second, the string of a tampon provides some support to the vaginal walls and the pelvic floor muscles. This can also help to prevent prolapse. If you are concerned about prolapse, or if you have already been diagnosed with prolapse, talk to your doctor about whether or not using a tampon is right for you.

Overall, the pelvic floor is an important muscle group that can impact a person's quality of life. While many people may not be familiar with the term, most are familiar with common problems that can arise when the pelvic floor muscles are weak or damaged. These problems can include incontinence, prolapse, and sexual dysfunction. Fortunately, there are many things that can be done to improve the strength and function of the pelvic floor muscles, including exercise, diet, and weight management. By paying attention to the health of the pelvic floor, both men and women can enjoy a better quality of life.

Can you be intimate with a prolapse?

A prolapse happens when one or more organs in the pelvis slip down from their original position and protrude into the vagina. Depending on the severity of the prolapse, penetration during intercourse may not be possible. In less severe cases, a prolapse may only make penetration uncomfortable. If the prolapse is severe, it may prevent intercourse altogether.

Assuming the article is discussing the pelvic floor in women: The pelvic floor is a group of muscles, ligaments, and connective tissue that supports the organs in the pelvis (bladder, uterus, and rectum). These muscles and tissues can weaken with age, pregnancy, and childbirth, which can lead to urinary incontinence and other problems. Pelvic floor exercises (such as Kegels) can help to strengthen the pelvic floor and improve its function.

Can a prolapse burst?

When most people think of a prolapse, they think of it as something that can happen to an organ like the uterus or bladder. However, the prolapse can also affect the pelvic floor. The pelvic floor is made up of the muscles and tissues that support the organs in the pelvis. When these muscles and tissues are weakened, they can no longer support the organs, and the organ may prolapse, or fall out of place. The pelvic floor can be weakened by many things, including pregnancy, childbirth, aging, and being overweight. When the pelvic floor is weakened, the organs it supports are no longer held in place as well as they used to be. This can cause the organs to sag or bulge, and in some cases, prolapse. A prolapse can happen slowly over time, or it can happen suddenly. Sometimes, a prolapse can happen after a sudden event, like coughing or lifting something heavy. Other times, a prolapse can happen gradually, and the person may not even know it's happening. Most prolapses are not painful, but they can be uncomfortable. A person with a prolapse may feel like they need to pee more often, or they may feel pressure in their pelvis. In some cases, a prolapse can cause pain, or make it difficult to have a bowel movement. If a prolapse is not treated, it can get worse over time. In some cases, a prolapse can become so severe that the organ falls out of the body entirely. This is rare, but it can happen. If this happens, it is a medical emergency, and the person needs to go to the hospital right away. A prolapse can be treated with surgery, but in many cases, it can be treated without surgery. If the prolapse is mild, a doctor may recommend lifestyle changes, like losing weight or avoiding constipation. A doctor may also recommend doing pelvic floor exercises to strengthen the muscles and tissues around the organs. In some cases, a doctor may insert a device called a pessary into the vagina to support the organs. Surgery is usually only recommended for severe prolapses, or for prolapses that are getting worse. The type of surgery will depend on the organ that is prolapsing. For example, if the uterus is prolapsing, a surgeon may do a hysterectomy, which is a surgery to remove the uterus. Most prolapses can be treated without surgery, but it is important to see a doctor if you think you may have a prolapse. A prolapse is not something that will go away on its own, and it can get worse over time. If you have a prolapse, there are treatment options available, and you don't have to live with it.

The pelvic floor is an incredibly important muscle group that supports the organs in the pelvis and helps to control urinary and bowel function. Unfortunately, this muscle group is often neglected in both men and women, which can lead to weak pelvic floors and incontinence. However, there are treatments and exercises available to help strengthen the pelvic floor. With the proper attention and care, the pelvic floor can be a strong, supportive muscle group.

How do you get rid of a prolapse without surgery?

A prolapse is when your pelvic organs drop down from their normal position and bulge into your vagina. They can also bulge into your anus (rectal prolapse) or outside of your body (labeled as an external prolapse). Prolapses are usually caused by a combination of factors, including: -weakening of the tissues that support your pelvic organs -pregnancy and childbirth -being overweight or obese -chronic coughing or sneezing -constipation -age-related changes in your tissues and muscles There are many different types of prolapse, but the most common are uterine, rectal, and bladder prolapse. Most prolapses can be treated without surgery. The goal of treatment is to relieve your symptoms and stop the prolapse from getting worse. Treatment options include: -pelvic floor muscle exercises -vaginal pessary -hormone therapy -weight loss - avoidance of constipation Pelvic floor muscle exercises, also called Kegel exercises, help to strengthen the muscles that support your pelvic organs. A vaginal pessary is a small, soft device that is inserted into your vagina to support your pelvic organs. Hormone therapy can be used to treat prolapse caused by menopause. Weight loss can help to reduce the pressure on your pelvic organs. Avoiding constipation can also help to reduce your symptoms. If your prolapse is severe or not responding to other treatments, surgery may be recommended. Surgery is usually only considered for severe prolapse that is causing serious symptoms. The type of surgery will depend on the type of prolapse you have. Uterine prolapse is usually treated with a hysterectomy (removal of the uterus). Rectal prolapse is usually treated with rectopexy (a surgery to attach the rectum to the pelvis). Bladder prolapse is usually treated with a sacrocolpopexy (a surgery to attach the bladder to the pelvis).

How do I know if my prolapse is severe?

Prolapse is a condition where the organs of the pelvis region fall down or slip out of place. This can be a result of pregnancy, childbirth, menopause, or simply due to the natural aging process. Many women experience prolapse and don't even know it because it often doesn't create any symptoms. However, in some cases, prolapse can be severe and cause significant discomfort. There are three main types of prolapse: 1. Rectal prolapse: This is when the rectum drops down into the anal canal or sticks out through the anus. 2. Bladder prolapse: This is when the bladder droops down into the vagina. 3. Uterine prolapse: This is when the uterus slips down into the vagina. If you are experiencing any of the following symptoms, it is important to see a doctor to determine if you have a prolapse: 1. Fever 2. Pelvic pain 3. Pain during intercourse 4. difficulty urinating or having a bowel movement 5. A bulge or protrusion in the vagina 6. Leaking urine or stool 7. Feeling like you are going to faint or collapse 8. Recurrent urinary tract infections If you are diagnosed with a prolapse, there are several treatment options available depending on the severity of your condition. In some cases, a simple change in lifestyle habits, such as managing your weight or avoiding constipation, can help to ease symptoms and improve your condition. For more severe cases, there are various surgical options available to correct the prolapse. No matter how severe your prolapse is, it is important to seek medical attention if you are experiencing any of the symptoms listed above. By catching the condition early, you can start treatment and reduce your risk of complications.

What is a stage 3 prolapse?

A stage 3 prolapse is when the pelvic organs (bladder, uterus, or rectum) have descended so far that they protrude out of the vagina. This can cause incontinence, pain during intercourse, and difficulty emptying your bladder or bowels. A stage 3 prolapse is a serious condition that requires treatment.

If you have a pelvic floor disorder, you're not alone. Over 17 million women in the United States suffer from some type of pelvic floor disorder.

And while pelvic floor disorders can happen to anyone, they are most common in women who have had children. There are many different types of pelvic floor disorders, but the most common are urinary incontinence and pelvic organ prolapse. Urinary incontinence is the involuntary leakage of urine and can happen when you cough, sneeze, or even laugh. Pelvic organ prolapse happens when the organs in your pelvis (uterus, bladder, or rectum) drop down from their normal position and protrude into the vagina. While there is no cure for pelvic floor disorders, there are treatments that can help. If you suffer from urinary incontinence, there are many different types of medication and devices that can help you manage your symptoms. Pelvic organ prolapse can be treated with surgery, but there are also many different exercises that can help strengthen the pelvic floor muscles and provide support for the organs. No matter what type of pelvic floor disorder you have, there are treatments available to help you manage your symptoms and improve your quality of life.

What causes a vaginal prolapse?

A vaginal prolapse occurs when the tissues and muscles supporting the vagina weaken and stretch, causing the vagina to sag or fall into the vaginal canal or out of the body. The most common cause of vaginal prolapse is childbirth, although it can also be caused by other factors such as menopause,hysterectomy, or being overweight.

Does a prolapse happen suddenly?

A prolapse happens when the pelvic floor muscles weaken and can no longer support the pelvic organs. The organs then drop down and may protrude through the vaginal opening. A prolapse can happen suddenly, but usually it develops slowly over time. There are several reasons why the pelvic floor muscles may weaken. Childbirth is a common cause, especially if the baby is large or delivered vaginally. Other causes include being overweight, having a chronic cough, and lifting heavy objects. Symptoms of a prolapse vary depending on the organs involved. A rectal prolapse, for example, may cause rectal bleeding or a feeling of pressure in the rectum. A vaginal prolapse may cause discomfort during sex, difficulty urinating, or problems with bowel movements. prolapse can also cause a feeling of fullness or pressure in the pelvic area. A prolapse is usually diagnosed through a physical exam. The doctor will look for bulges or protrusions in the vaginal area. They may also perform a pelvic Exam or an ultrasound to get a better view of the pelvic organs. Treatment for a prolapse depends on the severity of the condition. In some cases, the prolapse can be treated with lifestyle changes, such as losing weight or avoiding activities that put strain on the pelvic floor. If these changes don't help, there are several surgical options. The most common surgery for a prolapse is a pelvic floor repair. This surgery involves placing stitches in the muscles and tissues to support the pelvic organs.

At what stage of prolapse require surgery?

Prolapse is a medical condition that occurs when organs in the pelvis slump or drop down from their original position. The pelvic organs include the bladder, uterus, and rectum. These organs are supported by the pelvic floor, a group of muscles and ligaments that stretch like a hammock from the pubic bone to the tailbone. When the pelvic floor muscles are weak or damaged, they can no longer support the organs, and prolapse occurs. There are different degrees of prolapse, and not all prolapses require surgery. In some cases, mild prolapse can be treated with lifestyle changes, such as avoiding heavy lifting, constipation, and coughing. Kegel exercises, which strengthen the pelvic floor muscles, may also be recommended. If these conservative measures don't improve the prolapse, or if it's severe, surgery may be necessary. The type of surgery will depend on the organs involved and the severity of the prolapse. For example, a vaginal prolapse may be treated with a simple surgical procedure to insert a supportive device, called a pessary, into the vagina. A more serious prolapse may require surgery to remove excess tissue and repair the pelvic floor muscles. Prolapse is a common condition, particularly after childbirth or in older women. If you're experience prolapse, talk to your doctor about the best treatment options for you.

What can be mistaken for prolapse?

There are a few conditions that can be mistaken for prolapse. One is endometriosis, which is the growth of uterine tissue outside of the uterus. This can cause pain and bulging in the pelvic area. Another condition is fibroids, which are non-cancerous growths in the uterus. Fibroids can also cause pain and bulging in the pelvic area. Ovarian cysts can also cause pain and bulging in the pelvic area. However, ovarian cysts are usually not related to prolapse.

What is the most common organ to prolapse?

The most common organ to prolapse is the uterus. Other organs that may prolapse are the bladder, rectum, or small bowel. Symptoms of organ prolapse vary depending on the severity of the prolapse. Mild prolapse may not cause any symptoms. More severe prolapse may cause pressure or pain in the pelvic area, difficulty passing stool or urinating, or problems with sexual function. Organ prolapse is most often caused by pregnancy and childbirth. Other risk factors include obesity, chronic coughing, and constipation. Treatment for organ prolapse often involves lifestyle changes, such as weight loss and avoiding constipation. Surgery may also be necessary to repair the prolapse.

Are squats good for prolapse?

When it comes to prolapse, there are a lot of different opinions on whether or not squats are good. Some say that they are great for strengthening the pelvic floor, while others claim that they can actually make the prolapse worse. So, what is the truth? There is no doubt that squats are a great way to strengthen the muscles around the pelvis, including the pelvic floor muscles. However, there is no evidence to suggest that they can actually reverse or prevent prolapse. In fact, if you already have prolapse,squats may actually make it worse. This is because when you have prolapse, your pelvic organs are already drooping down into the vaginal canal. Doing squats puts a lot of pressure on these organs, which can cause them to drop down even further. Additionally, if you have prolapse, you may already have weak pelvic floor muscles. Doing squats puts a lot of strain on these muscles, which can lead to even further weakness and prolapse. If you are struggling with prolapse, it is important to talk to your doctor about the best exercises for you. They may recommend specific exercises that can help to strengthen your pelvic floor muscles and reduce the pressure on your pelvic organs. However, they will likely advise against doing squats. While there is no evidence that squats can help with prolapse, there are many other exercises that can. If you are struggling with prolapse, talk to your doctor about which exercises are best for you.

What is the best sleeping position for pelvic organ prolapse?

Pelvic organ prolapse is a condition in which the organs in the pelvis slip down from their normal position and bulge into the vagina. This can happen when the muscles and ligaments supporting the organs weaken or loosen. It is most common after menopause, but it can also happen after childbirth, with certain types of surgery, or with certain medical conditions. There are different types of pelvic organ prolapse, depending on which organs are affected. The most common type is uterine prolapse, which happens when the uterus slips down into the vagina. Other types of prolapse include ovarian prolapse (when the ovaries slip down), vaginal prolapse (when the walls of the vagina collapse), and rectal prolapse (when the rectum bulges into the vagina). There are several things that can help prevent or treat pelvic organ prolapse. One of the most important is to maintain a healthy weight. overweight and obesity are a major risk factor for prolapse, so losing weight if you are overweight or obese can help reduce your risk. Another important factor is to avoid chronic constipation. Constipation can put pressure on the pelvic organs and cause them to prolapse. To avoid constipation, eat a high-fiber diet and drink plenty of fluids. If you are already constipated, ask your doctor about laxatives or stool softeners. There are also a number of pelvic floor exercises that can help to strengthen the muscles and ligaments supporting the pelvic organs. These exercises are often called Kegel exercises, and they can be done anywhere, at any time. To do a Kegel exercise, simply squeeze the muscles you would use to stop the flow of urine. Hold the squeeze for a few seconds, then release. Repeat this 10-15 times, 3-4 times per day. Finally, one of the best things you can do for your pelvic health is to quit smoking. Smoking is a major risk factor for all types of prolapse, so quitting will help reduce your risk. There is no one "best" sleeping position for people with pelvic organ prolapse. However, lying on your back with a pillow under your knees can help take the pressure off of your pelvic organs and may help to reduce symptoms. Other positions, such as lying on your side or sitting up, may also be helpful. Experiment to see what position is most comfortable for you.

The pelvic floor is an essential part of the female anatomy, and it's important to keep it healthy and strong. There are a number of ways to do this, including exercise, Kegel exercises, and avoiding constipation. By taking care of your pelvic floor, you can help prevent issues like incontinence and prolapse.

What are 4 types of urinary incontinence?

There are four primary types of urinary incontinence: stress incontinence, urge incontinence, overflow incontinence, and functional incontinence. Stress incontinence is the involuntary leakage of urine during activities that put pressure on the bladder, such as coughing, sneezing, laughing, or exercise. This type of incontinence is often caused by weak pelvic floor muscles or damage to the nerves that control the muscles. Urge incontinence, also called overactive bladder, is a sudden, intense urge to urinate followed by an involuntary leakage of urine. This type of incontinence can be caused by a variety of factors, including medications, infection, nerve damage, and, in some cases, an overactive bladder muscle. Overflow incontinence is the constant or frequent leakage of urine due to a full bladder. This type of incontinence is often caused by an obstruction in the urinary tract, such as an enlarged prostate or a bladder stone. Functional incontinence is the leakage of urine due to a physical or mental impairment that prevents a person from making it to the toilet in time. This type of incontinence can be caused by a variety of factors, including arthritis, Parkinson's disease, stroke, and dementia.

How do you fix urinary incontinence?

The pelvic floor is the group of muscles and ligaments that support the bladder and other organs in the pelvis. A strong pelvic floor is essential for preventing urinary incontinence, which is the involuntary leakage of urine. There are a number of things that can weaken the pelvic floor, including pregnancy, childbirth, obesity, heavy lifting, and constipation. Pelvic floor exercises, also known as Kegels, are the most effective way to strengthen the pelvic floor. To do a Kegel exercise, tighten the muscles that you would use to stop the flow of urine. Hold the contraction for five seconds, and then relax for five seconds. Repeat this 10 times. If incontinence is a problem, there are a number of things that can be done to help. First, try to identify and avoid the activities or positions that make the problem worse. For example, if coughing or sneezing causes leakage, then coughing and sneezing should be avoided. Second, make sure to empty your bladder before participating in activities that may cause leakage. This will help to prevent leakage by minimizing the amount of urine in the bladder. Third, practicing Kegel exercises regularly can help to strengthen the pelvic floor muscles and decrease leakage. Finally, wearing absorbent pads or underwear can help to protect your clothing from urine leakage.

What are 3 treatment options for incontinence?

Pelvic floor incontinence is often treated with a combination of medical and lifestyle changes. Some common treatment options include: 1. Kegel exercises: These exercises strengthen the pelvic floor muscles, which can help to prevent or control incontinence. 2. Pelvic floor muscle training: This type of therapy uses exercises and electrical stimulation to help strengthen the pelvic floor muscles. 3. Biofeedback: This technique uses sensors to help people become aware of and control their pelvic floor muscle contractions. 4. Medications: There are a variety of medications that can be used to treat incontinence, depending on the underlying cause. 5. Surgery: In severe cases, surgery may be necessary to treat incontinence.

Does urinary incontinence go away?

Urinary incontinence is a common and often embarrassing problem. It is estimated that one in four women will experience some degree of urinary incontinence at some point in their lives. The good news is that urinary incontinence is often a treatable condition. There are many different types of urinary incontinence and the treatment will vary depending on the type and severity of the incontinence. In some cases, the incontinence may go away on its own. For example, stress incontinence is often seen during pregnancy and usually resolves after the baby is born. Other types of incontinence, such as overactive bladder, are more chronic and may require medical treatment. If you are experiencing urinary incontinence, it is important to talk to your doctor. He or she can help determine the cause of your incontinence and recommend the best treatment option for you.

What triggers incontinence?

There are many different factors that can contribute to incontinence. Sometimes it can be the result of a physical issue, such as a weak pelvic floor. Other times, it can be the result of a neurological condition, like Parkinson's disease. Still other times, it can be the result of a side effect from a medication. And sometimes, the cause of incontinence is unknown. There are many different things that can trigger incontinence episodes. Some people may find that they leak when they cough, sneeze, or laugh. Others may leak when they exercise or lift something heavy. For some people, incontinence may be related to a change in their diet or fluid intake. And, for some people, incontinence may happen when they're under a lot of stress. The most important thing to remember is that you're not alone. Incontinence is a very common issue, and there are many different treatments available. If you're struggling with incontinence, talk to your doctor. They can help you find the cause of your incontinence and develop a treatment plan that will work for you.

What are the first signs of incontinence?

There are a few key things to look for when it comes to the first signs of incontinence. Most importantly, pay attention to any changes in your bathroom habits. This can include anything from needing to go more frequently to struggling to make it to the bathroom in time. pelvic floor weakness may also cause you to leak a small amount of urine when you cough, sneeze, or laugh. Another early sign of incontinence is feeling like you can't completely empty your bladder. This can lead to urinary retention, which is when urine becomes stored in the bladder and doesn't get released. This can cause a number of uncomfortable symptoms, like pain in the lower abdomen and a feeling of fullness in the bladder. If you're experiencing any of these symptoms, it's important to talk to your doctor. They can help you figure out what's causing your incontinence and come up with a treatment plan.

Will drinking more water help with urinary incontinence?

Urinary incontinence is a common problem, especially among women. While there are many possible causes, one of the most common is weak pelvic floor muscles. These muscles support the bladder and help to keep it closed. When they are weak, the bladder can leak urine. Drinking more water will not directly strengthen the pelvic floor muscles. However, it can help to relieve some of the symptoms of incontinence. When the body is properly hydrated, the urinary system does not have to work as hard. This can reduce the frequency of leaks. Additionally, water can help to dilute the urine and reduce the risk of UTIs. While drinking more water is not a cure for incontinence, it can be a helpful tool in managing the condition.

Pelvic floor dysfunction can be a debilitating and embarrassing condition, but it is also treatable. With the help of a knowledgeable and experienced pelvic floor physical therapist, many people with pelvic floor dysfunction can find relief and learn to manage their symptoms.

What is a good home remedy for incontinence?

There are a variety of home remedies that can help with incontinence. Some of the most popular ones include: -Exercising the pelvic floor muscles regularly. This can be done by doing simple exercises like clenching and releasing the muscles multiple times a day. -Avoiding foods and beverages that can irritate the bladder. This includes things like caffeine, alcohol, and spicy foods. -Doing relaxation techniques like yoga or meditation. This can help to ease stress and tension, which can sometimes be a trigger for incontinence. -Limiting the amount of fluids you consume in a day. This can help to prevent the need to urinate frequently, which can often be a trigger for incontinence. -Making sure to empty your bladder completely when you go to the bathroom. This can help to prevent leakage later on. If you are struggling with incontinence, it is important to talk to your doctor. There are a variety of treatments that can help, and the best one for you will depend on the underlying cause of your incontinence.

What is the most effective treatment for incontinence?

The most effective treatment for incontinence may vary depending on the individual. However, the most common and effective treatments are pelvic floor muscle training, bladder training, and medications. Pelvic floor muscle training is a type of physical therapy that strengthens the muscles of the pelvic floor. This can help to improve or even eliminate incontinence. Bladder training is another type of physical therapy that helps to retrain the bladder muscles. This can help to reduce the number of times you need to urinate, and can also help to reduce incontinence. Medications can also be effective in treating incontinence. There are a variety of medications available, and your doctor can help you to choose the one that is right for you.

What can a GP do for incontinence?

There are a number of things that your GP can do in order to help you with your incontinence. They will first want to make sure that there is no underlying medical condition that is causing your incontinence. Once they have ruled this out, they can provide you with advice and information on how to manage your incontinence. This may include lifestyle changes, such as losing weight or stopping smoking. They can also prescribe medication, such as anticholinergics, to help treat your incontinence. If your incontinence is severe, they may refer you to a continence advisor or urologist for further treatment.

How do doctors treat incontinence?

When treating incontinence, doctors will first look at the underlying cause. If the cause is a physical issue, such as a muscle weakness, they will work on strengthening the muscles. If the cause is a medication side effect, they will work with the patient to find a different medication. If the cause is an underlying health condition, they will treat the condition. There are also a few different types of treatments that can be used to help with incontinence. One type of treatment is behavioral therapy. This type of therapy can help patients learn to control their bladder muscles. Another type of treatment is electrical stimulation. This type of treatment uses electrical pulses to help the muscles of the pelvic floor to contract. In some cases, surgery may be necessary to treat incontinence. One type of surgery is a sling procedure. This type of surgery is used to support the urethra. Another type of surgery is a colposuspension. This type of surgery is used to lift the bladder neck and urethra.

What vitamin helps with bladder control?

The best vitamin for bladder control is Vitamin D. Vitamin D helps to strengthen the muscles in the bladder, which can help to prevent incontinence. Vitamin D can be found in foods such as fatty fish, eggs, and fortified milk. You can also get Vitamin D from supplements or exposure to sunlight.

What is average age of incontinence start?

Stress incontinence is the involuntary leakage of urine during physical activity such as coughing, laughing, or sneezing. It is the most common type of incontinence in women and is most often the result of weakening of the muscles and tissues that support the bladder. The average age of incontinence onset is 50 years old. However, it is important to note that stress incontinence can occur at any age. It is more common in women who have had children, as the muscles and tissues of the pelvic floor can be stretched and weakened during pregnancy and childbirth. There are a number of factors that can contribute to the onset of stress incontinence. These include: -Pregnancy and childbirth -Weakening of the pelvic floor muscles with age -Chronic coughing -Obesity -Surgery on the bladder, uterus, or rectum If you are experiencing stress incontinence, it is important to see your healthcare provider. They can help to determine the cause and recommend treatment options.

What happens if incontinence is left untreated?

Untreated incontinence can lead to a number of serious health problems. One of the most common problems is skin irritation. This is because when urine leaks onto the skin, it can cause moisture to build up. This moisture can then lead to the growth of bacteria, which can cause the skin to become irritated. Another problem that can occur if incontinence is left untreated is urinary tract infections. These occur when bacteria enters the urinary tract, and can cause a number of uncomfortable symptoms, such as pain when urinating, a frequent need to urinate, and cloudy urine. If left untreated, urinary tract infections can lead to kidney damage. untreated incontinence can also lead to social isolation. This is because many people with incontinence feel embarrassed about their condition, and may avoid social situations for fear of having an accident. This can lead to a decline in mental health, as well as a decrease in overall quality of life. If you are experiencing incontinence, it is important to talk to a medical professional. There are a number of treatments available that can help to manage the condition, and prevent the serious health problems that can occur if it is left untreated.

The pelvic floor is an integral part of the female body and its function is to support the weight of the abdominal organs, as well as to control the release of urine and feces. When the pelvic floor muscles are weak, they can no longer effectively support the organs and may cause incontinence or prolapse. Pelvic floor exercises can help to strengthen these muscles and improve the function of the pelvic floor.

When should I see a doctor about incontinence?

There are a number of different factors that can contribute to incontinence, and often times the cause isn't clear. If you've been unable to control your urinary leakage for more than a month, it's time to make an appointment to see your doctor. Keep in mind that incontinence is not a normal part of aging, so don't hesitate to bring it up with your physician. Your doctor will want to get a full picture of your symptoms in order to make an accurate diagnosis. Be prepared to answer questions about how often you leak, what triggers your leaks, how much urine you leak each time, and whether you're also experiencing any urinary urgency or frequency. Your doctor will also likely want to rule out any potential medical causes of incontinence. This may involve ordering tests such as a urine analysis, bladder diary, post-void residual measurement, urodynamic testing, or cystoscopy. Once any underlying medical conditions have been ruled out or treated, your doctor may recommend pelvic floor muscle exercises and/or behavioral changes to help you manage your incontinence. In some cases, medications or surgery may be necessary. If your incontinence is particularly bothersome or interfering with your quality of life, don't hesitate to bring it up with your doctor.

Why can't I hold my pee all of a sudden as a woman?

There are a number of reasons why a woman may suddenly find herself unable to hold her urine. One possibility is that she has developed what is known as urinary incontinence. This is a condition in which the muscles that support the bladder are weak or have become damaged, making it difficult to control urination. Incontinence can be caused by a variety of things, including childbirth, menopause, and certain medical conditions. Another possibility is that the woman has a urinary tract infection (UTI). This is an infection of the urinary system, and can cause a strong and sudden urge to urinate. UTIs are often treated with antibiotics. Finally, it is possible that the woman is simply drinking too much fluid. If she is drinking a lot of water or other fluids, her body will need to get rid of it eventually and she may feel an urge to urinate more often than usual.

Is incontinence a symptom of stress?

Stress is a common cause of incontinence. When you're stressed, your body goes into "fight or flight" mode. This causes your body to release stress hormones, which can lead to muscle tension and increased heart rate. This can also lead to problems with sphincter control, which can cause incontinence. Incontinence is also a common symptom of anxiety disorders. People with anxiety disorders may have trouble controlling their urination or bowel movements. This can be due to muscle tension or changes in brain chemistry. Incontinence can also be caused by physical problems, such as an overactive bladder, weak muscles, or nerve damage. This type of incontinence is more common in older adults. If you're experiencing incontinence, it's important to see a doctor to rule out any physical causes. Once physical causes have been ruled out, you can work with a mental health professional to address stress and anxiety.

Can incontinence be repaired?

The pelvic floor is a group of muscles and tissues that stretch from the pubic bone to the tailbone. It supports the bladder and helps to control urination. Urinary incontinence is the leakage of urine. It can be a bothersome problem, but it is not usually a sign of a serious health problem. Overactive bladder, stress incontinence, and urge incontinence are the three main types of urinary incontinence. There are many treatments for urinary incontinence. The best treatment depends on the type of incontinence, its severity, and the underlying cause. Often, a combination of treatments is effective. Some of the most common treatments for urinary incontinence are: - Pelvic floor muscle exercises: These exercises can help to strengthen the muscles that support the bladder and help to control urination. - Absorbent products: These products, such as pads and liners, can help to absorb urine and protect clothing from leakage. - Medications: There are several medications that can be used to treat urinary incontinence. These include anticholinergics, beta-3 agonists, and tricyclic antidepressants. - Bladder training: This involves retraining the bladder to hold urine for longer periods of time. - Surgery: In some cases, surgery may be necessary to treat urinary incontinence.

What makes incontinence worse?

There are a number of things that can make incontinence worse. For example, if you are overweight, this can put extra pressure on your pelvic floor muscles and make them weaker. This can also be the case if you have had a baby – the added strain on your muscles can cause them to weaken and lead to incontinence. Constipation can also make incontinence worse, as it can put pressure on your pelvic floor muscles and lead to them becoming weaker. This is because when you are constipated, you often have to strain to go to the toilet, which puts extra pressure on your pelvic floor. Coughing and sneezing can also cause incontinence, as they put extra pressure on your pelvic floor muscles. This is because when you cough or sneeze, your pelvic floor muscles have to work hard to keep your bladder and bowel from emptying. If you have any type of pelvic floor surgery, this can also weaken your muscles and lead to incontinence. This is because surgery can damage the nerves and muscles in your pelvic floor. Finally, certain medications can also lead to incontinence. For example, some treatments for overactive bladder can cause incontinence. In addition, some antidepressants and blood pressure medications can also cause incontinence.

What not to drink when you have incontinence?

When it comes to incontinence, what you drink can be just as important as what you don't drink. Too much liquid can obviously lead to more trips to the bathroom, but did you know that certain drinks can actually irritate your bladder and make your symptoms worse? Here are four beverages to avoid if you're struggling with incontinence. Coffee. You may not want to hear this, but that morning cup of joe could be exacerbating your incontinence. Coffee is a diuretic, which means it makes you have to pee more. It also contains caffeine, which is a bladder irritant. If you're struggling with incontinence, it's best to cut back on coffee or switch to decaf. Tea. Like coffee, tea is also a diuretic. However, some types of tea may be worse than others. For example, green tea contains caffeine, while herbal tea may contain bladder-irritating herbs such as juniper or parsley. If you enjoy tea, stick to decaffeinated varieties. Soda. If you're struggling with incontinence, you may want to stay away from soda. Not only is it full of sugar, which can irritate your bladder, but it also contains caffeine, which as we've mentioned, is a bladder irritant. Alcohol. You may have heard that alcohol can help to relax the muscles, but when it comes to your bladder, that's not necessarily a good thing. Alcohol can actually lead to urinary incontinence because it relaxes the muscles that control urine flow. So, if you're struggling with incontinence, it's best to avoid alcohol or at least limit your consumption. If you're struggling with incontinence, it's important to be mindful of what you're drinking. While you don't necessarily have to give up your favorite beverages entirely, you may want to limit your consumption or switch to decaf or decaffeinated varieties.

Which medications cause incontinence?

There are many potential medications that could potentially cause incontinence. These medications can include, but are not limited to, those used to treat high blood pressure, Parkinson's disease, Alzheimer's disease, and seizures. bladder-controlling medications, sedatives, and certain antidepressants. These medications work by affecting the muscles and nerves that control urination. When these muscles and nerves are affected, it can cause incontinence. There are many different medications that can cause incontinence, so it is important to speak to a doctor if this is a concern. Incontinence can be a difficult and embarrassing condition to deal with, but there are treatments available.

The pelvic floor is an important group of muscles, ligaments, and connective tissue that supports the organs in the pelvis and helps to keep them in place. pelvic floor dysfunction can cause a wide variety of problems, including incontinence, sexual dysfunction, and pain. Pelvic floor dysfunction is a common problem, but it is often underdiagnosed and undertreated. There are a variety of treatments available that can help to improve symptoms and quality of life.

How long does incontinence last?

Incontinence is a symptom, not a disease, and it can last for a variable amount of time. Some people only experience incontinence for a short time after an event that causes undue stress on the pelvic floor, such as childbirth, surgery, or an injury. For others, incontinence may be a chronic problem. There are many factors that can contribute to the duration of incontinence. Pelvic floor muscle strength and tone play a role in supporting the bladder and bowel. When these muscles are weakened, incontinence may result. Other factors that can influence the duration of incontinence include the type and severity of the incontinence, overall health, and age. There are many different types of incontinence, each with its own set of causes and treatments. The most common types of incontinence are urinary incontinence and fecal incontinence. Urinary incontinence is the involuntary leakage of urine. It can be caused by a number of things, including weakened pelvic floor muscles, damage to the nerves that control the bladder, and certain medications. Fecal incontinence is the involuntary leakage of stool. It can be caused by damage to the nerves that control the bowel, or by muscle damage or weakness in the pelvic floor or anal sphincter. Incontinence can be a temporary or chronic problem. If incontinence is a temporary problem, it is often due to a specific event or situation, such as childbirth, surgery, or an injury. If incontinence is a chronic problem, it may be due to a more underlying condition, such as an neurological disorder, diabetes, or a weakened pelvic floor. There are many treatments available for incontinence, and the best course of treatment will vary depending on the individual and the type and severity of incontinence. Some people may only need brief treatments, such as lifestyle changes or pelvic floor muscle exercises, while others may require more long-term treatments, such as medication or surgery. Incontinence is a common problem, affecting millions of people of all ages. While it can be a nuisance, there are treatments available that can help to improve the condition.

Does incontinence get worse with age?

There's no simple answer to whether incontinence gets worse with age. While it's true that the condition is more common in older adults, there are a number of factors that can contribute to incontinence and its severity. Age itself isn't necessarily a cause of incontinence. But as we get older, our bodies change in ways that can make incontinence more likely. For example, older adults are more likely to have weakened muscles and reduced muscle tone. This can make it harder to hold in urine or feces. Similarly, the aging process can cause changes in the nerves that control the urinary and anal sphincters. These changes can make it difficult to know when to urinate or defecate, and can also lead to leakages. There are a number of underlying health conditions that can also contribute to incontinence. These include diabetes, Parkinson's disease, and multiple sclerosis. In addition, certain medications can cause incontinence or make it worse. These include diuretics, sedatives, and certain types of antidepressants. Incontinence can also be a side effect of certain medical procedures, such as a radical prostatectomy. There are a number of lifestyle factors that can increase the risk of incontinence or make it worse. These include being overweight or obese, smoking, and drinking alcohol. While incontinence is more common in older adults, it is not a normal part of aging. If you are experiencing incontinence, it is important to talk to your doctor. There are a number of treatments available that can help to improve the condition.

What is the first line of treatment for urinary incontinence?

The first line of treatment for urinary incontinence is pelvic floor muscle training. This is a form of exercise that strengthens the muscles around the bladder and urethra, which helps to prevent leakage. The exercises can be done at home, and there are many resources available to help you get started. If you have leakage that is severe or persistent, you may need to see a doctor or other healthcare provider to find out what other treatments are available.

Does magnesium help with incontinence?

Magnesium is a mineral that is important for many processes in the body, including muscle function. Some people believe that magnesium can help to treat incontinence, although there is not much scientific evidence to support this claim. Magnesium is involved in muscle contraction and relaxation. This means that it could potentially help to relax the muscles in the pelvic floor, which could help to prevent incontinence. However, there is no scientific evidence to support this claim. There are some studies that have looked at the effects of magnesium supplements on incontinence. One study found that magnesium supplementation improved symptoms of stress incontinence in postmenopausal women. However, this study had a small number of participants and more research is needed to confirm its findings. Another study found that magnesium was no more effective than a placebo in treating urge incontinence. This study also had a small number of participants and more research is needed to confirm its findings. Overall, there is not enough scientific evidence to say that magnesium definitely helps with incontinence. However, it is a safe supplement to take and it may help some people. If you are thinking about taking magnesium supplements for incontinence, it is important to speak to a doctor or other healthcare professional first.

What drinks are good for your bladder?

When it comes to bladder health, what you drink matters. drinks like caffeine and alcohol are diuretics, which means they make you have to urinate more. This can lead to dehydration, which can irritate the bladder. Carbonated drinks can also lead to bladder problems because they can cause gas and bloating, which puts pressure on the bladder. So what should you drink? Water is the best choice for keeping your bladder healthy. It's calorie-free, caffeine-free, and sugar-free. It also helps to keep your body hydrated, which is important for overall health. Drink plenty of water throughout the day, and make sure to urinate regularly. Other good choices for drinks include: -herbal teas -fruit juices -soups Drinking these liquids can help to flush out bacteria and keep the bladder clean. Cranberry juice is also a good choice, as it is rich in natural antioxidants and can help to fight infection. If you're experiencing bladder problems, it's best to avoid diuretics and carbonated drinks. Stick to water and other healthy liquids, and see your doctor if you're still having problems.

What is the best sleeping position for overactive bladder?

The best sleeping position for overactive bladder may vary from person to person. Some people may find that sleeping on their back allows gravity to keep their bladder in place, while others may find that sleeping on their side or stomach keeps their bladder from bulging and pressing against the mattress. Ultimately, the best sleeping position for overactive bladder is the position that is most comfortable for the individual and allows them to sleep through the night without waking up to use the restroom.

Can you be incontinent and not know it?

It's estimated that one in three women will experience incontinence at some point in their lives. For some, it's a occasional drippy situation. Others may leak a little when they jump, laugh, or sneeze. Still, others feel as if they've totally lost control and are constantly running to the bathroom. Because there's such a range of severity, it's possible to have incontinence and not even know it. Here's the thing: A little bit of leakage is considered normal. In fact, research has found that up to 20% of women may experience what's known as stress urinary incontinence (SUI), which is when urine leaks out during activities that put pressure on the bladder, like coughing, sneezing, and jumping. The good news is that there are treatments available that can help with SUI. But what about those women who are constantly leaking? This is where things can get a bit more complicated. There are a number of different types of incontinence, and each one has its own set of causes and treatments. For example, Urge incontinence, which is also called Overactive Bladder, occurs when the muscles in the bladder contract too often, causing a sudden, urgent need to urinate. This can be caused by a number of things, including medications, infection, and nerve damage. Then there's Functional incontinence, which is when an underlying condition makes it difficult to get to the bathroom in time. This can be due to things like arthritis, Parkinson's disease, or Stroke. There are also a number of other less common types of incontinence, including: - Overflow incontinence: This is when the bladder doesn't empty completely and urine leaks out. - Mixed incontinence: This is when a person experiences more than one type of incontinence. - Transient incontinence: This is a temporary form of incontinence that can be caused by things like medications, constipation, or urinary tract infection. If you're constantly leaking urine, it's important to talk to your doctor. They can help you figure out what's causing your incontinence and come up with a treatment plan.

The pelvic floor is an important part of the human body. It supports the internal organs and prevents them from prolapsing. It also helps to control the flow of urine and feces. Pelvic floor dysfunction can cause a variety of problems, including incontinence, prolapse, and sexual dysfunction. Pelvic floor exercises can help to strengthen the muscles and prevent dysfunction.

How do they fix female urinary incontinence?

The pelvic floor is a layer of muscle and connective tissue that supports the bladder, uterus, and rectum. It also helps to control the release of urine and stool. When the pelvic floor is weakened, it can lead to problems with urinary or fecal incontinence. There are a variety of treatments for urinary incontinence in women. The type of treatment that is best for you will depend on the causes and severity of your incontinence. Some of the most common treatments for urinary incontinence include: Pelvic floor muscle exercises: These exercises can help to strengthen the muscles around the bladder and urethra. This can help to improve or even cure stress incontinence. Weight loss: Being overweight can put extra pressure on the bladder and urethra. Losing weight can help to reduce this pressure and improve incontinence. Avoiding bladder irritants: Certain foods and drinks can irritate the bladder and make incontinence worse. Avoiding these irritants can help to improve your symptoms. Bladder re-training: This treatment involves learning to control when you urinate. You will work with a health care provider to set a schedule for urination and gradually increase the time between bathroom visits. Medications: There are a variety of medications that can be used to treat urinary incontinence. These medications can help to relax the bladder muscles, reduce urinary urgency, or increase the amount of urine your body can hold. Injections: A chemical called botulinum toxin (Botox) can be injected into the bladder muscle. This can help to reduce bladder spasms and improve incontinence. Surgery: In some cases, surgery may be recommended to treat urinary incontinence. Surgical options include sling procedures, artificial urinary sphincter, and bladder neck suspension. No matter what treatment you choose, it is important to remember that incontinence is a treatable condition. With the help of a health care provider, you can find the treatment that works best for you.

Should I be worried if I can't hold my pee?

If you are unable to hold your urine, it is important to consult with a doctor to rule out any underlying medical conditions. There are a number of conditions that can cause urinary incontinence, such as a weak pelvic floor, bladder prolapse, or nerve damage. While some of these conditions can be treated, others may require more long-term management. There are also a number of lifestyle factors that can contribute to urinary incontinence, such as diet, weight, and exercise. Urinary incontinence is a common problem, affecting up to one in three women. While it can be embarrassing and inconvenient, it is important to remember that you are not alone. There are a number of treatments available to help manage urinary incontinence. If you are worried about your urinary incontinence, speak to your doctor for advice.

How do you fix bowel incontinence?

There are a number of ways that you can fix bowel incontinence, and the best way will vary depending on the individual case. In some cases, changes to your diet may be enough to fix the problem. For example, if you are eating too much fiber, cutting back on the amount of fiber you consume may help to fix the problem. Other times, more drastic measures may be necessary. For example, if changes to your diet do not help, you may need to have surgery to repair the damage to your digestive system. This is usually only necessary in extreme cases, however. In most cases, bowel incontinence can be fixed with a combination of dietary changes, medication, and exercises to strengthen the muscles in your pelvic floor. With the proper treatment, most people are able to control their bowel incontinence and live relatively normal lives.

What causes bowel incontinence?

There are many different conditions that can cause bowel incontinence. In some cases, it may be a result of a physical problem, such as an injury to the anal sphincter (the muscle that controls bowel movements). Other times, it may be due to a neurological disorder, such as multiple sclerosis or Parkinson's disease. Bowel incontinence can also be a side effect of certain medications, such as those used to treat diarrhea, constipation, or depression. In some cases, it may be a symptom of a more serious underlying medical condition, such as cancer or inflammatory bowel disease. often, the exact cause of bowel incontinence is unknown. However, there are certain risk factors that can make a person more likely to experience the condition, such as being female, having had a baby, being older, or having a family history of incontinence.

What are the 4 types of bowel incontinence?

There are four types of bowel incontinence: 1. Urine incontinence: This is the inability to control urination. 2. Fecal incontinence: This is the inability to control bowel movements. 3. Sphincter incontinence: This is when the muscles that control the opening and closing of the anus are unable to function properly. 4. Gastrointestinal incontinence: This is when the stomach muscles are unable to function properly.

How do you stop bowel incontinence naturally?

There are a number of things you can do to stop bowel incontinence naturally. The most important thing is to make sure that you are getting enough fiber in your diet. This will help to make your stools softer and easier to pass. You should also make sure that you are drinking plenty of fluids, as this will help to keep your stools from becoming too hard. Another important thing to do is to make sure that you are exercising regularly. This will help to keep your muscles strong and healthy, which will in turn help to keep your bowel movements regular. If you are having trouble getting enough exercise, there are a number of ways to make it easier, such as taking the stairs instead of the elevator, or parking further away from your destination. In addition to dietary and lifestyle changes, there are a number of supplements that can help to stop bowel incontinence. Probiotics are one type of supplement that can be particularly helpful, as they help to restoring the balance of bacteria in the gut. Other supplements that may be helpful include fiber supplements, such as psyllium husk, and anti-spasmodic herbs, such as chamomile and ginger.

When should I be concerned about bowel incontinence?

Bowel incontinence, also called fecal incontinence or anal incontinence, is the accidental passing of solid or liquid stool. It can be a very embarrassing and distressing problem. While occasional episodes of bowel incontinence are not a cause for concern, persistent or frequent bowel incontinence may be a sign of a more serious underlying medical condition. If you are experiencing persistent or severe bowel incontinence, it is important to see your doctor for a proper diagnosis and treatment. There are a number of different causes of bowel incontinence. Common causes include: - Weak anal sphincter muscles: The anal sphincter is a ring of muscle that helps to keep stool in the rectum. If the anal sphincter muscle is weak, it may not be able to hold back stool, leading to incontinence. - Damaged anal sphincter muscles: The anal sphincter muscle can be damaged by childbirth, surgery, or other trauma. This can lead to incontinence. - Diarrhea: Diarrhea can cause incontinence by making it difficult to control the passing of stool. - Constipation: Constipation can make incontinence worse by hardening the stool and making it difficult to pass. - Neurological conditions: Conditions such as stroke, spinal cord injury, or multiple sclerosis can damage the nerves that control the anal sphincter muscles. This can lead to incontinence. Treatment for bowel incontinence will vary depending on the underlying cause. In some cases, such as with constipation, treatment may be as simple as making lifestyle changes, such as eating a high-fiber diet and drinking plenty of fluids. In other cases, more aggressive treatment may be necessary, such as medication, biofeedback, or surgery. If you are experiencing bowel incontinence, it is important to see your doctor for a proper diagnosis and treatment. Treatment can help to improve your quality of life and may help to prevent serious complications, such as skin infections.

The pelvic floor is a group of muscles, ligaments, and connective tissue that form a hammock-like structure at the base of the pelvis. These muscles and tissues support the pelvic organs, including the bladder, uterus, and rectum, and help to control bowel and urinary function. Pelvic floor dysfunction can cause a number of problems, including incontinence, prolapse, and sexual dysfunction. Fortunately, there are treatments available to help improve pelvic floor function and relieve symptoms.

Is bowel incontinence life threatening?

No, bowel incontinence is not life threatening. However, it can have a significant impact on a person's quality of life. The condition can cause embarrassment and social isolation, and can also lead to skin infections and dehydration. There are a number of treatments available for bowel incontinence, and the type of treatment will depend on the underlying cause of the condition. In some cases, the incontinence can be managed with dietary changes, medications, or pelvic floor muscle training. In more severe cases, surgery may be required. If you are experiencing bowel incontinence, it is important to speak to your doctor to discuss your symptoms and find the best treatment option for you.

Can faecal incontinence be cured?

Around one in three people experience faecal incontinence at some point in their lives. For some, it is a short-term problem that can be cured. However, for others, it may be a lifelong condition. There are a number of treatments that can be effective for faecal incontinence. These include dietary changes, medication, bowel training and surgery. Dietary changes: Making some simple changes to your diet can be effective in treating faecal incontinence. This includes avoiding foods that can make your stool loose, such as spicy food, cheese and caffeine. Eating more fibre can also help to firm up your stool. Medication: There are a number of different types of medication that can be used to treat faecal incontinence. This includes anti-diarrhoeal medication, which can help to firm up your stool. There are also medications that can help to reduce muscle spasm and inflammation. Bowel training: Bowel training can be an effective treatment for faecal incontinence. This involves retraining your bowel muscles to help them work properly. This can be done through a number of different exercises, such as Kegel exercises. Surgery: In some cases, surgery may be required to treat faecal incontinence. This can be done to repair damage to the anal sphincter muscles. Surgery can also be used to create an artificial anal sphincter.

Why do I constantly wipe after bowel movement?

When you have a bowel movement, your pelvic floor muscles relax to allow your bowels to empty. After you finish going to the bathroom, these same muscles contract, or squeeze, to close off your rectum and anus. If your pelvic floor muscles are weak, they may not be able to fully contract. This can cause stool to leak from your rectum, which can be both embarrassing and uncomfortable. You may also feel the need to constantly wipe after bowel movements because there is stool remaining in your anus. There are a number of things that can weaken your pelvic floor muscles, including pregnancy, childbirth, and aging. Overweight and obese people are also more likely to have weak pelvic floor muscles. Fortunately, there are exercises you can do to strengthen your pelvic floor muscles. These exercises, which are sometimes called Kegel exercises, can be done anywhere and at any time. They don't require any special equipment, and you can do them sitting, standing, or lying down. If you're not sure how to do Kegel exercises, talk to your doctor or pelvic floor physical therapist. They can give you instructions and guidance so that you can be sure you're doing them correctly.

What is it called when you can t control your bowel movements?

The act of losing control of one's bowels is known as fecal incontinence. This can be a very embarrassing and difficult problem to deal with. There are many causes of fecal incontinence, including; - damage to the muscles or nerves around the rectum or anus - changes in diet - chronic constipation - diarrhea Fecal incontinence is often treated with a combination of lifestyle changes, dietary modification, and medications. In some cases, surgery may be necessary. If you are struggling with fecal incontinence, it is important to talk to your doctor to determine the best course of treatment for you.

How common is bowel leakage?

It's estimated that 1 in 3 women experience some form of bowel leakage. For some, it's a occasional leaks during moments of laughter or physical exertion. But for others, it's a chronic condition that can have a significant impact on quality of life. There are a number of factors that can contribute to bowel leakage. Women who have had childbirth are more likely to experience it, as are those who have had certain surgeries involving the pelvis or gastrointestinal tract. Obesity and chronic constipation can also increase the risk. While there's no shame in talking about bowel leakage, it can be a tough subject to broach with your doctor. But it's important to do so, as there are treatments available that can help. In some cases, making simple lifestyle changes like eating a high-fiber diet and getting regular exercise can make a big difference. In other cases, medication or surgery may be necessary. If you're dealing with bowel leakage, know that you're not alone. With the right treatment, you can often manage the condition and enjoy a good quality of life.

How do I tighten my sphincter muscle?

The pelvic floor is a group of muscles and ligaments that support the bladder, bowel, and uterus. The pelvic floor muscles are located between the pubic bone and the tailbone. The pelvic floor muscles play an important role in urination, defecation, and childbirth. The pelvic floor muscles can be weakened by pregnancy, childbirth, surgery, and aging. The best way to tighten the pelvic floor muscles is to do pelvic floor muscle exercises (also called Kegel exercises). To do pelvic floor muscle exercises: 1. Find the right muscles. The best way to find the right muscles is to stop urination in midstream. The muscles you use to do this are the pelvic floor muscles. 2. Squeeze the muscles. Once you have found the right muscles, squeeze them for 3 to 5 seconds, and then relax for 5 seconds. 3. Repeat. Repeat this exercise 10 to 15 times. You can do pelvic floor muscle exercises anywhere and anytime. You don't need any special equipment. You can do them sitting, standing, or lying down. If you're having trouble doing pelvic floor muscle exercises, you can try using a vaginal cone or weight. A vaginal cone is a small, weighted device that you insert into the vagina. You can also use a pelvic floor muscle toner. A pelvic floor muscle toner is a small, battery-operated device that sends gentle electrical pulses to the pelvic floor muscles. These devices are available without a prescription. If you are doing pelvic floor muscle exercises and you are not sure if you are doing them correctly, you can ask your doctor or pelvic floor physical therapist to check you.

What foods can cause bowel incontinence?

There are a variety of foods that can cause bowel incontinence, and it is important to be aware of which foods may trigger an episode. Some common offenders include highly processed foods, fried foods, Dairy products, caffeine, alcohol, and artificial sweeteners. Highly processed foods are often hard to digest, and can cause abdominal pain and bloating. Fried foods are also difficult to digest, and can cause abdominal pain and cramping. Dairy products can cause diarrhea, and caffeine can act as a diuretic, causing loose stools. Alcohol can also cause diarrhea. Artificial sweeteners can cause gas and bloating. Eating a balanced diet is important for overall health, but it is especially important for people with bowel incontinence. Eating a diet that is low in fiber can make the condition worse. Fiber helps to bulk up the stool and makes it easier to pass. Foods that are high in fiber include fruits, vegetables, beans, and whole grains. Drinking plenty of fluids is also important for people with bowel incontinence. Fluids help to keep the stool soft and easy to pass. Water is the best fluid to drink, but juices and decaffeinated teas can also be helpful. It is important to avoid caffeine, as it can act as a diuretic and make the condition worse. If you have bowel incontinence, it is important to talk to your doctor about which foods may trigger your symptoms. There is no one-size-fits-all diet for people with bowel incontinence, but avoiding trigger foods and eating a diet that is high in fiber and fluids can help to manage the condition.

The pelvic floor is a group of muscles and ligaments that support the bladder, uterus, and rectum. These muscles and ligaments can be weakened by childbirth, aging, and obesity, resulting in urinary incontinence, pelvic organ prolapse, and fecal incontinence. Kegel exercises are one way to strengthen the pelvic floor.

How can I prevent bowel incontinence in old age?

As we age, our bodies change in a variety of ways. One such change is a weakening of the pelvic floor muscles. These muscles play an important role in bowel control, and a weakened pelvic floor can lead to incontinence. There are a number of things you can do to prevent or reduce the likelihood of bowel incontinence in old age. First, it's important to maintain good bowel habits. This means regular, soft, and easy-to-pass stools. Constipation puts unnecessary strain on the pelvic floor muscles and can lead to leakage. Secondly, you can perform exercises to strengthen the pelvic floor muscles. These exercises, known as Kegels, can be done anywhere and at any time. Simply squeeze the muscles you would use to stop the flow of urine, and hold for 10 seconds. Repeat this 10 times, 3 times per day. Finally, it's important to maintain a healthy weight. Excess weight puts strain on the pelvic floor muscles, and can lead to incontinence.

Losing weight can be difficult, but even a modest weight loss can improve bowel control. By following these simple tips, you can help prevent bowel incontinence in old age.

Is bowel incontinence a normal part of aging?

As we age, our bodies go through a lot of changes. Some of these changes are normal, and others can be a sign of disease or injury. When it comes to bowel incontinence, there is a lot of misunderstanding about what is normal and what is not. Bowel incontinence is the involuntary leakage of stool. It can happen to anyone, at any age, but is more common in older adults. There are many different causes of bowel incontinence, and it is important to see a doctor to rule out any serious medical conditions. Age-related changes in the body can contribute to bowel incontinence. These include changes in muscle tone, nerve function, and stool consistency. Some medications can also cause or worsen incontinence. Incontinence is not a normal part of aging, but it is a common problem. If you are experiencing incontinence, talk to your doctor. There are many treatments available that can help you manage your symptoms and regain control of your bowel.

What cancers cause bowel incontinence?

Cancer can cause bowel incontinence in several ways. First, cancer can directly invade and damage the muscles and nerves of the pelvic floor that control bowel function. Second, cancer can indirectly cause bowel incontinence by damaging the central nervous system (CNS) or autonomic nervous system (ANS), which control bowel function. Third, cancer can cause inflammation or obstruction of the bowel, which can lead to incontinence. There are many different types of cancer that can cause bowel incontinence. The most common are colorectal cancer, anal cancer, and rectal cancer. Other cancers that can cause bowel incontinence include bladder cancer, ovarian cancer, and prostate cancer. Cancer that directly invades the pelvic floor muscles and nerves is the most likely to cause bowel incontinence. The pelvic floor muscles control the function of the anal sphincter, which is a muscular ring that keeps the anal canal closed. The anal sphincter muscles relax to allow solid waste to pass through the anal canal and contract to keep the anal canal closed. When the pelvic floor muscles are damaged by cancer, the anal sphincter muscles may not work properly, leading to incontinence. Cancer that damages the CNS or ANS can also cause bowel incontinence. The CNS controls the function of the digestive system through the brain and spinal cord. The ANS controls the function of the digestive system through the nerves that connect the brain and spinal cord to the digestive organs. damage to either the CNS or the ANS can disrupt the normal function of the digestive system and lead to incontinence. Cancer-related inflammation or obstruction of the bowel can also cause incontinence. Inflammation is the response of the body to injury or infection. Cancer-related inflammation can damage the muscles and nerves of the pelvic floor and lead to incontinence. Obstruction occurs when something blocks the normal passage of bowel contents through the digestive system. Cancer can cause obstruction by growing into or narrow the passages of the digestive system. Obstruction can also be caused by the accumulation of scar tissue in the digestive system.

How do you know if you have bowel incontinence?

There are a few things that may help you know if you have bowel incontinence. One is if you have leakage of stool. This could be a small amount of stool leakage when you have a bowel movement, or it could be a large amount of leakage that occurs without you even having a bowel movement. Another thing that may help you know if you have bowel incontinence is if you have trouble control your bowel movements. This means that you may have a hard time knowing when you have to have a bowel movement, or you may have a lot of urgency before you have a bowel movement. You may also have a feeling that you need to have a bowel movement but nothing comes out when you try. If you have any of these symptoms, it is important to talk to your doctor. They will be able to help you determine if you have bowel incontinence and help you find the best treatment for you.

Why do I get skid marks no matter how much I wipe?

When it comes to skid marks in your underwear, it could be a number of things. It could be that you are not wiping well enough, you could have a medical condition, or you may be eating foods that are difficult to digest. If you are not wiping well enough, it is important to make sure that you are wiping from front to back. This will help to prevent any feces from getting into your urinary tract and causing an infection. If you are using a wipes, make sure that you are using one that is alcohol-free and gentle. You may also want to try using a moist toilet paper to help remove any residue. If you have a medical condition, it is important to talk to your doctor about any potential links to skid marks. Some conditions, such as celiac disease, can cause chronic diarrhea which can lead to skid marks. IBS (Irritable Bowel Syndrome) is another condition that can cause skid marks. If you have any other medical conditions, be sure to speak with your doctor to rule out any possible causes. You may also be eating foods that are difficult to digest. Foods that are high in fiber can cause issues with digestion and may lead to skid marks. It is important to eat a balanced diet and to drink plenty of fluids to help with digestion. If you think that your diet may be the cause of your skid marks, you may want to speak with a dietitian to help you make some changes.

How far should you wipe after pooping?

When it comes to wiping after pooping, there is no one-size-fits-all answer. It depends on a variety of factors, including the type of stool, the amount of stool, and your own personal wiping preferences. If you have a soft stool, you may only need to wipe once or twice. If you have a more formed stool, you may need to wipe three or four times. And if you have a very loose or watery stool, you may need to wipe five or more times. The key is to wipe until your paper is clean. If you find yourself having to wipe more than five times, you may want to rethink your diet or talk to a doctor, as this could be a sign of a digestive issue. And when it comes to the actual wiping, be sure to wipe from front to back. This will help prevent the spread of bacteria from your anus to your vagina or urinary tract.

How long should you wipe after pooping?

There is no one-size-fits-all answer to this question, as the amount of time you spend wiping after a bowel movement will depend on a number of factors, including the size and consistency of your stool, the sensitivity of your skin, and the strength of your pelvic floor muscles. If you have a large, bulky stool, it is likely that you will need to spend more time wiping than someone with a smaller, softer stool. This is because there is more surface area to clean, and it can be more difficult to remove all traces of the stool without causing irritation. Similarly, if you have sensitive skin, you may need to be more careful when wiping, as harsh toilet paper can cause irritation and bleeding. In this case, it is often best to use a softer toilet paper, or even baby wipes. Finally, the strength of your pelvic floor muscles will also affect how long you need to spend wiping after a bowel movement. If your pelvic floor muscles are weak, you may need to spend more time wiping in order to prevent accidents, as these muscles help to control the flow of stool. Ultimately, there is no set amount of time that you should spend wiping after a bowel movement - it will depend on your individual circumstances. However, if you are taking longer than a few minutes to wipe, or if you are experiencing discomfort or irritation, it is worth speaking to a doctor or other healthcare professional to rule out any underlying conditions.

The pelvic floor is a group of muscles and ligaments that support the bladder, uterus, and rectum. The pelvic floor muscles are important for urine control, sexual function, and childbirth. Pelvic floor dysfunction can cause problems with urination, sexual function, and pelvic pain.

What are the best pads for faecal incontinence?

The best pads for faecal incontinence will vary depending on the individual's needs and preferences. Some factors to consider when choosing a pad include: the level of absorbency required, the size and shape of the pad, the length of time it needs to be worn, and the price. There are many different brands and types of pads available on the market, so it is important to do some research to find the best option for the individual. Online forums and reviews can be a helpful resource when choosing a pad. It is also important to talk to a healthcare professional to get specific recommendations.

What kind of doctor do you see for bowel incontinence?

Depending on the severity of your bowel incontinence, you may be able to manage the condition at home with lifestyle changes, such as diet modification and toilet routines. If your incontinence is more severe, you may need medication or surgery. In either case, you should start by talking to your primary care physician. If you have frequent or severe episodes of bowel incontinence, you may need to see a specialist, such as a gastroenterologist, colorectal surgeon, or urogynecologist. A gastroenterologist is a doctor who specializes in the digestive system. A colorectal surgeon specializes in surgery of the colon and rectum. A urogynecologist is a doctor who specializes in treating problems with the pelvic floor. Your primary care physician can refer you to a specialist if they feel it is necessary. You can also ask for a referral from friends or family, or you can search for a specialist in your area. Once you have found a specialist, you will need to schedule an appointment. During your appointment, the specialist will ask you about your symptoms and medical history. They may also perform a physical exam. In some cases, you may need to have a pelvic floor muscle assessment, which is a test to assess the strength and coordination of the muscles around the anus and rectum. After the initial assessment, the specialist will develop a treatment plan for you. If your incontinence is mild, you may only need to make lifestyle changes, such as changing your diet or using the toilet differently. If your incontinence is more severe, you may need medication or surgery. Medication There are several types of medication that can be used to treat bowel incontinence, including anti-diarrheal medication, stool softeners, and laxatives. Anti-diarrheal medication can help to reduce the frequency of bowel movements. Stool softeners can help to make stool easier to pass. Laxatives can help to increase the amount of water in the intestine, which can make stool softer and easier to pass. Surgery In some cases, surgery may be necessary to treat bowel incontinence. Surgery can be used to repair damage to the anal sphincter or to remove blockages in the intestine.

How do you know if your sphincter is damaged?

There are a few things that can happen that might indicate that your sphincter is damaged. One is if you feel like you can't hold in your bowel movements anymore and are losing control of your bowels. This would likely be accompanied by other symptoms like leakage or soiling of your undergarments. You might also have fecal incontinence, which is when gas or stool leaks from your rectum even when you don't want it to. Another symptom of a damaged sphincter is persistent pain in your anus or rectum. This pain might happen when you're having a bowel movement or afterwards. It can also happen even when you're not doing anything and just sitting or standing. The pain might be a sharp, burning sensation or a dull, aching feeling. If you think you might have a damaged sphincter, it's important to see a doctor so they can diagnose the problem and recommend treatment. Treatment options will vary depending on the cause and severity of the damage, but might include lifestyle changes, medication, surgery, or a combination of these.

Can a loose sphincter muscle be repaired?

A loose sphincter muscle can be repaired, but it may take some time and effort. The sphincter is a ring of muscle that helps to keep stool and gas from leaking out of the rectum. When the sphincter muscle is loose, it can allow stool and gas to leak out, which can be embarrassing and inconvenient. There are a few things that can cause the sphincter muscle to become loose, including pregnancy, childbirth, age, and obesity. The good news is that a loose sphincter muscle can be repaired. The first step is to see your doctor to find out if you have a loose sphincter muscle. Your doctor can do a digital rectal exam or an anorectal manometry to check for a loose sphincter muscle. If your doctor finds that you have a loose sphincter muscle, they will likely recommend lifestyle changes and pelvic floor exercises. Lifestyle changes that can help to improve a loose sphincter muscle include quitting smoking, losing weight if you are overweight, and avoiding constipation. Pelvic floor exercises, also called Kegel exercises, can also help to strengthen the sphincter muscle. To do a pelvic floor exercise, squeeze the muscles that you would use to stop the flow of urine. Hold the squeeze for 10 seconds, and then relax for 10 seconds. Repeat this exercise 10 times. If lifestyle changes and pelvic floor exercises do not improve a loose sphincter muscle, your doctor may recommend surgery. Surgery to repair a loose sphincter muscle is called an anal sphincteroplasty. During this surgery, the surgeon will make an incision in the anal sphincter muscle and sew it back together. This surgery is usually done as an outpatient procedure, which means you will not need to stay in the hospital overnight. A loose sphincter muscle can be repaired, but it may take some time and effort. The important thing is to talk to your doctor if you are having any problems with leakage of stool or gas. With the help of your doctor, you can make lifestyle changes and do exercises that can improve your condition.

What are the symptoms of a weak sphincter muscle?

When the pelvic floor muscles are weak, they cannot provide the same level of support to the pelvic organs as when they are strong. This can lead to a number of symptoms, such as: * Urinary incontinence: urine leaks when coughing, laughing, sneezing, or during exercise * Fecal incontinence: stool leaks when coughing, laughing, sneezing, or during exercise * Prolapse: the dropping down of pelvic organs such as the uterus, rectum, or bladder, into the vaginal canal * Pain during sex: because the pelvic organs are not being supported as they should be, they may be pushed down into the vaginal canal during intercourse, causing pain These symptoms can be embarrassing and cause a great deal of anxiety. They can also lead to a loss of sexual satisfaction and a decline in overall quality of life. If you are experiencing any of these symptoms, it is important to talk to your doctor. There are treatments available that can help to alleviate the symptoms and improve your quality of life.

Is bowel incontinence psychological?

It's a common question: can bowel incontinence be psychological? The answer is, it depends. If you're dealing with occasional leaks, then the answer is likely no. But, if you're struggling with chronic incontinence, there may be some psychological factors at play. For some people, bowel incontinence can be the result of psychological trauma, such as sexual abuse. This can lead to a condition called post-traumatic stress disorder (PTSD), which can cause incontinence. Other psychological conditions, such as anxiety and depression, can also lead to incontinence. stress and anxiety can lead to bowel incontinence by causing the muscles in the pelvic floor to tense up. This can make it difficult to hold in stool. Depression can also lead to incontinence by causing changes in brain chemistry that make it difficult to control the muscles in the pelvic floor. While psychological factors can certainly contribute to bowel incontinence, it's important to remember that there are many other possible causes, such as medical conditions, certain medications, and lifestyle factors. If you're struggling with incontinence, it's important to see a doctor so they can rule out any potential underlying causes.

The pelvic floor is a group of muscles that support the pelvic organs. These muscles can be weakened by pregnancy, childbirth, surgery, and other factors. A weak pelvic floor can lead to urinary incontinence and other problems. Kegel exercises are the best way to strengthen the pelvic floor muscles.

Is walking good for prolapse?

SD - #0046 - 140926 - C0 - 229/152/11 - PB - 9781776969449 - Matt Lamination